Health and Nursing Studies for
Diploma and Undergraduate Students

Health Ethics

by

Chris Henry and Glenys Pashley

\

Quay Publishing
11 Victoria Wharf
St George's Quay
Lancaster, LA1 1GA

British Library Cataloguing in Publication Data
Henry, Chris 1946-
    Health ethics – (Health and nursing studies for diploma and
    undergraduate students)
    1. Medicine. Ethical aspects
    I. Title II. Pashley, Glen 1955- III. Series
    174.2

    ISBN 1-85642-001-9

Health Ethics

**Health and Nursing Studies for
Diploma and Undergraduate Students**

Health Psychology
Authors: Glenys Pashley and Chris Henry
Health Ethics
Authors: Chris Henry and Glenys Pashley
Health Care Research
Authors: Chris Henry and Glenys Pashley

CONTENTS

Chapter 1
Introduction

a)   AIM OF THE COURSE TEXT

The aim of this study book for nurses on health care ethics is twofold: first to produce a text that is adequate in giving a good introduction to ethical knowledge and secondly to make difficult and obscure ethical concepts more available for application. The text has been originally designed to encourage different ways of thinking for the nurse. Ethics cannot give concrete answers but what it can do is help us to make more cautious and informed decisions in conflicting situations that arise within an increasingly advanced technological society.

The rapid changes occurring in nurse education emphasises the importance of the ethical domain for the new undergraduate and diplomate curricula. However, an appropriate text to complement the changes has not been a priority. The present authors, basing their claims on several years' experience of teaching both ethics and psychology to nurses and other health professionals, firmly believe that a course study text such as this is a priority and in one sense long overdue.

Each section of the text outlines major issues of concern for the nurse practitioner. Further, there are some suggested discussion questions which may help the student to utilise the process of theory into practice. The authors take the view that integration of theory into practice involves each unique individual cognitively assimilating and understanding major concepts, critically assessing and evaluating them, and having enough confidence to appropriately and sensitively utilise their thinking

1

processes to influence action. In other words, making informed decisions that influence and guide action and subsequently enhance better health care.

The book hopefully will encourage students to extend their grasp of theory into the nature of ethical practice and care. It does not involve a specific area of ethics such as nursing or medical ethics, but broad and diverse issues of applied ethics generally. Ethics, in this way, is viewed as a major domain of philosophical thought. The text is concerned with moving away from specific and personal philosophies and getting at the grass roots and foundations of nursing knowledge itself. It attempts to construct the beginnings of a philosophy of health care, a branch of inquiry which tries to analyse and understand the rationale of practice.

Seedhouse (1988) remarks that philosophies are concerned with the underlying reasons for the practical activities and consequently have an influence on the future development of them. The domain of applied health care ethics can certainly influence ethical practice but also health care and the evolution of a philosophy of nursing itself.

b)   WHAT IS HEALTH ETHICS?

It may be claimed that there are two major approaches to the study of morality. The first could be said to be scientific and descriptive and is often used within the social sciences. The social sciences deal with human behaviour and conduct but the emphasis is upon the empirical in that the sociologist or psychologist will observe and collect data about human behaviour and conduct and then try to draw conclusions. A developmental psychologist, for instance will, after observing and perhaps interviewing many children, reach the conclusion that there is a cognitive developmental trend in moral development. The developmental psychologist will subsequently try to develop a conceptual model and identify stages of moral development (see Piaget 1896–1980). This is a descriptive, and as some social scientists will claim, a scientific approach to the study of human behaviour. By contrast, the second approach to the study of morality is ethics and is distinct from this scientific way of understanding. What is important is to try to clarify the differences although it may be claimed that every scientific form of enquiry is still rooted in philosophy.

The second approach to the study of morality is the one upon which this text focuses and it can be divided into two appropriate parts:

1. The first part of this approach is opposite to the previous scientific or descriptive approach and is referred to as **normative** or **prescriptive** ethics. This form of ethical enquiry is to do with 'norms' and 'prescriptions' and goes far beyond the descriptions and conclusions of psychologists or sociologists. In this way the ethicist would want to know whether human beings, i.e. children and professional adults ought to be taught moral education at an early age in school or in their educational development. This is no longer merely a description but involves a prescription, i.e. an 'ought' and much more than an empirical or scientific enquiry because it involves values and normative concerns.

2. The second part of the ethical form of enquiry is called **meta ethics** or **analytical ethics**. These theorists concentrate on analysis, rather than prescriptiveness. They will analyse ethical language, for example, asking the question, "What do we mean by good?" The theorist may attempt an analysis of the rational foundations of an ethical system or logic and reasoning of various moral philosophers. (See Chapter 8, Two major perspectives of morality.) These theorists are not concerned with description, direct content or normative ethics.

A complete study of ethics demands the use of the descriptive, normative and meta ethical approaches and this is the underpinning intention of the present authors. The commitment involves some kind of **assimilation** and **synthesis** of understanding descriptive, normative and analytical ethics, with emphasis on creating an applied ethics useful in health care.

Ethics is concerned with the thought processes behind making moral judgements and based upon discussion of what is good, right and just. Further, it is worth bearing in mind that the two terms, ethics and morals, are used interchangeably and both refer to the issues of what is right and wrong in both theory and practice of human behaviour. Ethics and morality as terms are very significant in that the meaning and use enter into all our thoughts and actions as persons interacting with each other. Therefore, ethics may originate in every day life, and it would be a mistake to regard ethics as a purely academic study because it would, in one sense, be meaningless. Ethics has intimate connections with the daily lives of persons and every person who is reflective and troubled by certain situations in their professional and personal life is a philosopher of ethics.

Chapter 2
Reason and argument

ARGUMENT, REASON AND LOGIC

Philosophy is a highly argumentative discipline. Questions such as what constitutes current reasoning and what distinguishes a good argument from a bad one, are important for ethics. We produce reasons for reaching certain conclusions we wish to establish and these reasons allow us to infer conclusions. A person who has suitable reasons and arguments for what he/she says may well be described as being logical. Logic has also been used in a more technical sense as the science of reasoning where the structuring of an argument is placed within a formal system. Whilst this text will not be overtly concerned with formal logical systems, it may be useful to discuss briefly Aristotle's **Syllogism** (384–322 BC). This is the oldest formal system and it will give a basic introduction to a few logical terms that may be of use in the process of reasoning.

The oldest example states:

> "All men are mortal
> Socrates is a man
> Therefore, Socrates is mortal".

The first two statements of the syllogism are called **premises**. One argues from the premises. The final statement is the **conclusion**. These are used in all kinds of arguments (see moral arguments). Another major concept of importance in formal and informal arguments is that of **validity**. An argument may be claimed to be valid if the conclusion really does follow from the premises. It will be viewed as invalid if it does not follow from the premises. Nevertheless, it is important to point out that something being valid does not mean the same as something being true. A valid argument shows that the conclusion follows from the premises. The argument could be valid even though the premises are false, e.g.

> All nurses are wealthy.
> I am a nurse.
> Therefore I am wealthy.

The argument is valid but the first premise is not true, so the conclusion is not proved.

Moral arguments

Moral arguments have an underlying form in that there is a major premise (a moral rule or principle), a minor premise (a statement of fact connecting the situation under discussion with the rule) and a conclusion (what we ought or ought not to do).

e.g.   *Major premise.* One ought not to deceive a person about a matter which is important for her future health and welfare. *Minor premise.* Failure to disclose to Smith the full facts about her treatment deceives her about a matter which is important to her future health and welfare. *Conclusion.* Therefore (ergo), it is wrong not to disclose to Smith the full facts of her treatment. *Conclusion*

Discussion about the arguments can be either about the minor premise (the facts) or about the rule, (the major premise). The facts might be inaccurate, mistaken or incomplete, or they may not really apply to the rule. Discussion about the minor premise may involve questions of scientific knowledge. However, the discussion of the facts will often involve moral judgements, like whether or not there is full disclosure of the facts.

The major premise might again be moral, factual or conceptual although the emphasis will be on morality. For example it may be wrong to deceive people about matters affecting their own health and welfare but it is also wrong to give them information which will upset them at a crucial stage of their illness. (Other moral issues are brought in here, like person autonomy, paternalism etc.) In discussion about the major premise we connect our argument to higher order principles.

RELEVANCE AND MISCONCEPTIONS

Arguments are not always different from statements and the conclusion of one argument may serve as a premise in a second argument.

Knowledge of technical logic is not necessary and certainly not sufficient for arguments that link facts to values, i.e. in (some) moral arguments. Further, **deductive** arguments are much more common than **inductive** arguments within the moral domains. **Inductive** arguments are more common in the scientific, empirical or descriptive areas (see Chapter 1).

Deductive arguments are likely to be analytical, necessary or conceptual, for example "Bachelors are unmarried men." The definition is in the premise itself, i.e. the truth, which is necessary and analytical. By contrast, **inductive** arguments are usually linked to the empirical form of inquiry and are factual and contingent, for example "Most doctors play cricket." This is probably only based upon observation and, therefore, empirical only contingent and not necessary.

In all arguments it is important that the premises supporting the conclusion are of the appropriate kind.

FALLACIES

When an argument has the form of a syllogism and seems valid but is not, we say it is a fallacy. A fallacy is any sort of mistake in reasoning or inference. The following are some examples:

Fallacies of ambiguity: A term is ambiguous if it has more than one meaning, e.g.
> All men are brothers on a common fraternity.
> All brothers in a common fraternity are college students.
> All men are college students.

The word fraternity is used in two different senses.

Contextual fallacies: One of the most common is the fallacy of significance. Advertising claims often commit this fallacy, e.g.
> 62% of those doctors who smoke, smoke Goldies!

This is obviously misleading since it does not say how many doctors do not smoke, nor does it say that they smoke only Goldies!

Fallacy of emphasis: Self-evident, e.g.
> *Protection guaranteed against everything* except death, injury or disease

Fallacy of argumentum ad hominem: This is the most difficult to expose as well as being the most common. It is an argument directed against an individual rather than what the individual says, in order to show that what he/she says cannot be true, e.g.

> **Socialist:** It is essential that we limit nuclear tests because it may help to destroy our environment
>
> *Opponent:* *You cannot believe what she says, since she is a socialist and they always try to control military expenditure.*

A statement cannot be shown to be false merely because the individual who makes it can be shown to be a person of defective character.

Fallacy of appeals to sentiment: These attempt to establish that a given statement is true or false by reporting on how people feel about it, e.g.

It is wrong to have an abortion since that is what most people believe.

We cannot prove whether something is wrong or not by the beliefs of the majority of people.

Fallacy of the argumentum ad ignorantiam: This sort of argument contends that some statements must be true because there is no evidence to disprove them.

Fallacy of non-sequitur: Simply means it does not follow.

Finally, appeals to authority are not really worthy of moral debate. People in authority or who have expertise in a particular field may have better views on moral questions than the rest of us, but moral questions do not require expertise of that sort. A doctor who is an expert in medical matters and probably an excellent practitioner is not necessarily an expert in making moral decisions. Training/education does not prepare him/her in any way for claiming authority in making moral decisions. The fallacy of arguing from authority is a common type of fallacy but one cannot prove the truth or falsity of a given statement merely because someone in authority says so. It is not the prestige of an authority which makes a statement true or false but rather the citing of evidence either to confirm or refute the statement. Moral questions cannot be settled by appeals to authority and this is especially relevant in health care.

SUMMARY OF KEY POINTS

A.　i)　　Philosophy is an argumentative discipline
　　ii)　　What distinguishes a good argument from a bad one is crucial for ethics
　　iii)　　Reasons allow us to **infer** a **conclusion**
　　iv)　　A **syllogism** is the oldest formal system of logic
　　v)　　You argue from a **premise** to a conclusion
　　vi)　　An argument is **valid** if the conclusion follows from the premise
　　vii)　　An argument can be valid even though the premises are false

B.　i)　　Moral arguments have a **major premise** which is usually a moral rule or principle
　　ii)　　Moral arguments have a **minor premise** that may be a statement of fact connecting the situation under discussion with the major rule
　　iii)　　Moral arguments have a conclusion saying that we ought or ought not to do something
　　iv)　　The major premise might be (**moral**), **factual** or **conceptual**

C.　i)　　Knowledge of technical logic is not necessary or sufficient for arguments that link facts to values
　　ii)　　**Deductive** arguments are analytical, necessary or conceptual
　　iii)　　**Inductive** arguments are empirical, factual and contingent
　　iv)　　When an argument has the form of a syllogism and seems valid but isn't, it is called a **fallacy**
　　v)　　Appeals to authority are not worthy of moral debate

DISCUSSION QUESTIONS

1. Try to identify the major parts of an argument, recognising the major premises, the minor premises and the conclusion. Use any of the brief arguments in this section if you cannot construct your own.

2. Why is it that an argument can be valid but not true?

3. Explain why a deductive form of argument is different from the inductive form of argument.

4. What is a fallacy? Explain in your own words and try to give a specific example of the committing of a fallacy within the health care field.

5. "The doctor says that I ought not to tell Mrs Jones that her treatment can be extremely painful. The drugs have severe side effects but it is necessary that she is given the drugs in order to help her recover. The doctor believes that it would cause distress to Mrs Jones and, therefore, we must not tell her. I am accountable to the doctor. He has the authority, therefore, I must not tell Mrs Jones."
   Is there anything wrong with what this nurse is saying?

Chapter 3
Subjective and objective views

SUBJECTIVE VIEWS

If something is viewed as neither true nor false, it is seen as subjective. This is particularly true in relation to ethical judgements, for example, the statement "Mercy killing is wrong". The denial that moral beliefs and judgements are ever true or false is a version of subjectivism

The theory of **emotivism** contends that moral judgements are neither true nor false but merely expressive of feelings. If the emotivist theory is correct, it follows that moral judgements cannot be reduced to scientific ones. (See Chapter 1: What is Health Ethics? Two approaches to study morality...). The theory states that moral judgements are not analogous to scientific statements and that there is no assertion or description of anything. It means that moral judgements cannot be verified or · falsified by scientific procedures and that moral judgements are about one's feelings. They are the expression of feelings, much like a grunt of pleasure.

Values are often viewed as subjective, morality stemming from within human beings. In other words, we need a person or persons to put values on things and if there were no persons then there would be no values. Ethics deals with values, such as good, bad, right and wrong, and the question arises, "Are these values totally subjective?"

Fitzpatrick (1988) remarks that someone who expresses a moral viewpoint is reporting his own attitudes concerning the issue in question, e.g. abortion is wrong. What the person is saying is, "I disapprove of the acts of abortion. If I disapprove, then what I say is true." This brand of subjectivism treats moral beliefs and judgements as true or false but denies that they make any assertion about the nature of those acts. "The beliefs and attitudes report my own moral attitude." This type of subjectivism is different from the first type but is sometimes found in medicine and nursing.

Arguments for subjectivism

1. The main argument rests upon the analysis of the language that we use to make moral judgements. Those judgements are more than just statements or descriptions. They are imperatives and are prescriptive, evaluative and expressions of one's personal values. They have moral elements which are not descriptive and it does not make sense at all to ask whether they are true or false.

2. The argument from sentience remarks that we should imagine a world in which there were no creatures which had feelings, desires etc., no sentient beings in the world! The subjectivist says that it would not make sense to say that anything is good or bad or to ascribe such predicates. It is only sentient beings who affect these events. The subjectivist goes on to say that ultimately what is good or bad depends upon the individual psychology of the person.

3. The egoistic argument is used to reject objectivist theories such as utilitarianism. It says, "What is the point of working for the greatest happiness for the greatest number if you personally become unhappy by doing so. In the final analysis who can be more important than yourself. If a course of action leads to the well being of others but not yourself can it really be good?" The subjectivists say that we can only justify working for the good of many if it includes self.

13

Arguments against subjectivism

1. If we accept such a theory we can never settle any dispute. How can we say that Hitler was wrong if we accept subjectivism? All it would mean is that I disapprove of Hitler. If Hitler objected to this and claimed he did right by killing 6,000,000 Jewish persons then he would mean "I approve". There is no real conflict because both are talking about how they feel, not about the act of killing these people.

2. A second difficulty is that words like good, bad, right and wrong have more or less the same meaning for everybody in commonsense terms. If they did not, it would be impossible to communicate. These words must have some interpersonal meaning. However, with the subjectivist doctrine two different people would never mean the same thing when they utter these words. When I say something is good I am not only expressing my approval but also drawing attention to the fact that most people approve of it.

3. The third difficulty is that such subjectivist views cannot justify the concept of duty. In moral agony the notion of doing one's duty seems to involve acting against one's inclinations, at least some of the time. Subjectivist theories can explain such a concept if they reduce all moral behaviour to liking and disliking.

OBJECTIVE VIEWS

Values viewed as objective

There are two basic theories from which concepts of objective value arise: the natural theory and the supernatural theory. The natural theory indicates that others believe morality is somehow embodied in nature and that there are natural laws which human beings must adhere to if they are to be moral (St. Thomas Aquinas, 1225 – 1274). For example, some people will state that homosexuality is immoral because it goes against the natural morality, i.e. it is against the nature of beings of the same sex to love one another in a sexual sense. The supernatural theory indicates that values come from some higher order being or principle (the Good in Platonic doctrine, Jahweh or God for the Jews, Allah for the Muslims). They believe that these beings or principles embody the highest good in themselves and they reveal to human beings what is right or good. If human beings want to be moral they must follow the teachings of these beings or principles.

We can define the term objectivist by saying that any theory which is not subjectivist is objectivist.

Arguments against the objective position

Objectivists contend that there is no essential difference between a dispute about moral matters and a dispute about factual ones and one fact can be right and one can be wrong. Further, such theories can explicate the nature of duty by saying that duties are objective facts. The main difficulty centres around how we establish or prove that a certain action is right or wrong. This is the kind of difficulty that leads the subjectivists to believe that moral statements are not the same as scientific statements and therefore cannot have objectivity.

It is possible that the supernatural exists. However, it is only a belief based on faith and there is no conclusive proof. It is difficult to establish with certainty that morality comes from this source. We talk about laws of nature such as gravity, but they are quite different from man-made laws having to do with morality. Natural laws are descriptive whereas moral laws are prescriptive.

SUMMARY OF KEY POINTS

Subjective views

i)   If something is viewed as neither true nor false it is seen as subjective

ii)   Emotivism contends that moral judgements are neither true nor false but merely expressive of feelings

iii)   Moral judgements cannot be reduced to scientific ones

iv)   Values come from human beings. If there were no human beings there would be no values

v)   One's own attitudes express a moral view point in supporting "I disapprove of this act." This view point treats moral beliefs as true or false but denies that they make assertions about the nature of those acts

vi)   Subjectivism states that judgements are imperatives, prescriptive and evaluative. It does not make sense to ask if they are true or false

vii)   How can we accept subjectivism as a theory if we can never settle the dispute and say "Hitler was wrong"

viii) There is some similarity in meaning of words like good and bad in commonsense terms but not from the subjectivist position. Further, there is no room for the concept of duty or acting against one's inclinations

Objective views

i)   Morality is embodied in nature and there are natural laws which human beings must adhere to, e.g. "Homosexuality is unnatural"

ii)   The supernatural theory is that values come from a higher order being or principle

iii) How do we establish or prove a certain action is right or wrong by objective facts such as duty?

iv)   How can one establish that morality comes from a supernatural being or principle?

DISCUSSION QUESTIONS

1.   Are values totally subjective?

2.   Is it possible to have any natural moral laws?

3.   Can moral judgements ever be true or false? Discuss in relation to the objectivists position.

4.   Why is it that moral judgements are not the same as scientific ones?

5.   Why is it important for nurses and other health professionals to understand subjective and objective views in ethics?

Chapter 4
Absolute and relative views

Absolutists maintain that there are absolute truths, especially moral truths, to which persons must adhere to if they are to be moral.

Relativism maintains that there are no absolutes of any kind but everything, especially morality, is 'relative' to particular cultures, groups and individuals (Thiroux, 1977).

THE MEANING AND APPLICATION OF ABSOLUTE

Essentially, 'absolute' means perfect quality without limit by restrictions or exceptions and not to be doubted. It is unconditional and we apply it to supernatural beings, e.g. God or the universal good, to laws of nature, propositions, law and morality and truth. This links with the objectivist view.

Truth will apply to propositions which are meaningful statements describing states of affairs, occurrences and events. Propositions are either true or false, never states of affairs – they either occur or do not occur.

Truth is absolute and not relative to belief, knowledge, person, place or time. If propositions are stated accurately this will always hold.

There are several types of propositions:

1. Analytical propositions are truths which are known to be absolute, e.g. all triangles are three-sided

2. Internal sense or state propositions are propositions we know are true merely because we have the experience, e.g. I have a pain

3. Empirical or external sense propositions describe a state of affairs in the world of which we have evidence through our senses

4. Moral propositions are propositions about morality or moral import, e.g. persons should never kill other persons. These moral propositions are empirical and rational in form. Some philosophers say moral statements are not propositions at all in that they are merely emotive utterances (subjective and emotive theory). Some say that because they are not based on fact they cannot be true or false

The concept of absolutes is impossible to maintain because we still have the problem of matching propositions with the complexity of human thought, feeling and actions. To do this we must move from the concept of absolutes to that of 'near absolutes' or alternatively basic principles. A basic principle, because it approximates to an absolute, ought to be adhered to unless there is strong justification for not doing so.

RELATIVISM

It is important to distinguish at least three forms of relativism:

1. Descriptive relativism which simply states that the basic ethical beliefs and value judgements of different persons and societies are different and even conflicting

2. Meta ethical relativism which is the view that, in the case of basic ethical or value judgements at least there is no objectively valid rational way of justifying one against the other. Consequently two conflicting basic judgements may be equally valid

3. Normative relativism. Descriptive relativism makes anthropological or sociological assertions and meta ethical relativism makes a meta ethical assertion. This form of relativism puts forward a normative principle: what is right or good for one individual or society may not be right or good for another, even if situations are similar. However, such a normative principle violates the requirements for universalisation (see Chapter 8, under Kantian ethics, p48)

Some anthropological facts are cited in support of cultural relativism in that there are extreme variations in customs, manners, taboos and religions from culture to culture. Further, moral beliefs and attitudes of human beings are learned essentially from cultural environments. People in different cultures tend to believe that their morality is the one true morality.

Criticisms

Just because cultures differ about what is right and wrong does not mean that one culture is right and another is wrong. If beliefs are learned it does not mean that they are true or false or that truth is relative to specific societies. However, we still have to bear in mind that if moral principles are similar in all societies this does not mean that they are valid or absolute. Further, because there are similarities in cultural situations, it does not mean that these are the only morally correct situations.

There is one world and this applies as much to ethics as to any other form of discourse. We must accept that it is impossible to attain truth in any ultimate sense, or argue outside all conceptual frameworks. Ethics may or may not involve standards of truth or falsity as applied to moral judgements, as we may only talk in terms of correct or meaningful discourse. To be a relativist about value is to maintain that there are no universal standards of good and bad, right and wrong. To be a relativist about fact is to maintain that there is no such thing as objective knowledge of realities independent of the knower.

SUMMARY OF KEY POINTS

Absolutist views

i)   There are absolute truths about moral matters (objectivism)

ii)   It is unconditional and we can apply it to supernatural beings, i.e. God or to laws of nature

iii) Propositions are true or false and truth is absolute

iv)   The concept of absolutes is impossible to maintain. All we can do is approximate towards an ideal principle: 'a near absolute'

Relativist views

i)   We are concerned with normative relativism in that what is right or good for a person may not be good for another even if situations are similar

ii) This normative form of relativism has a meta ethical assertion of what is right or good but it violates the requirements for universalisation (see Chapter 8 under Kantian ethics, p48)

iii) Just because cultures differ about what is right and wrong does not mean that one culture is right and another is wrong

DISCUSSION QUESTIONS

1.   Is there a danger in nurses claiming that values are subjective and relative?

2.   Discuss how values may be both subjective and objective if we consider that there is something to value, a conscious agent who can value and a situation in which the valuing can take place.

3.   Try to define or explain the two terms **absolutist views** and **relativism**. Why would a nurse need to know about these two terms?

4.   Can truth be totally relative?

5.   Discuss why a nurse should adopt the basic principle of a **near absolute** unless she or he can justify an exception to it, e.g. "Always tell the patient or client the absolute truth."

Chapter 5
Persons

First, it is necessary to seek some understanding of what we mean by the concept of the 'person' and to whom we legitimately ascribe person status before discussing how important an understanding of the concept of persons and, subsequently, respect for persons may be for the nurse practitioner.

Persons

Abelson (1977) claims that the term 'person' is purely normative and evaluative like the term 'good', whilst the term 'human' is viewed as semi-normative and descriptive. The semi-normative element indicates aspects and characteristics that we value about humans, and links to the notion of how we use it in everyday commonsense ways, e.g. "Well, she's only human after all," indicating that there are human characteristics that are valued because we are human and not machine-like or perfect. However, the descriptive element of the term 'human' refers to species membership and is concerned with a natural description of a biological organism belonging to a species. The term 'person' on the other hand, is difficult to define or describe and is viewed as species neutral. In other words, it does not belong to a descriptive species category. According to Abelson the term 'person' is not a natural concept but an evaluative and moral concept. He states that neither logic nor language can solve the problem of who should and should not be counted as a person because it is an open-ended concept with moral and psychological features that are free from biological classification. Harris (1985) remarks that a person is any being capable of valuing its own existence. Midgley's response (1983) is that other animals besides ourselves may value their own existence and in this sense are capable of being persons. The problem surrounding Midgley's comment is that she assumes that we know that other animals have the ability to be self-reflective and rational.

Dennett (1979) proposes six necessary (but not sufficient) conditions of being a person. Although his list is open-ended, major person features include: ability to be rational, having intentions (psychological states of consciousness), the social aspect of being treated as a person and being able to reciprocate in some way, language and, finally, self-consciousness or self-reflection.

There is also an alternative way of understanding persons that links closely to a commonsense view. It is a view that Wittgenstein presents, avoiding attributing features to persons but understanding what we mean by the term person through the way we use language (Henry, 1986). An example can show how this may occur in everyday use of language. Further, it will highlight how the term 'human' and 'person' can be used interchangeably or have different meanings. A group of medical biologists may use the term 'human' to refer specifically to the biological species, whereas a group of nurses may use the term 'human' to refer to a 'person' when talking about a patient/client. The same word is used in each language game but has a different meaning.

The concept of the person, with some of its uses, stands for what humans essentially are, and more than one answer to what constitutes a person can be given. What appears to be important about people is that they are persons, not that they are of the same biological species. We treat humanity as the deciding mark for the ascription of personhood, not only because there are aspects of being human that are value laden, but because human beings are, so far, the only persons we recognise.

Moral issues for the concept of the person

It seems that the features applied to persons are neither perfectly rational nor clear cut. The term person is evaluative and moral, very much like the term 'good'. From an ethical standpoint we must assume that the term person is not only central to health care but is viewed as a moral term.

The point is that rights, justice and other ethical concepts do not apply to dealings and interactions of creatures that are not persons such as some other animals and machines. The term person is obviously not a natural term but a term created by persons themselves (Henry and Tuxill, 1987(b)).

Persons and non-persons

Some believe that the mentally handicapped, the very young infant and the foetus cannot be classed as persons. This question raises the ethical issues surrounding person/non-person distinctions for health care.

It seems that there are no clear natural dividing lines between some non-persons and persons (e.g. six-month foetus). It is the border-line cases that cause the problems.

In examining the concept of the person, several questions arise in relation to ethics of care and the assumption that **respect for persons** is central to health care. The distinction between persons and non-persons could depend upon whether the term person is meaningfully applicable or not. The foetus is human and a potential member of a rational species, but is it a person? Can it be inferred that the foetus, the severely defective child and the madly insane are in some way exempt from very important and crucial elements of personhood? Do we have a feature list and tick off what they have got? Alternatively, is it moral and open-ended or is the meaning in how we use the term?

Downie and Telfer (1980) point out that natural science explanations of the world are based upon conceptions of things. However, within the health care domains, it is essential to explore forms of knowledge more appropriately matched to conceptions of care. Ethics is one major applied domain that is essential, and part of the ethical curriculum should explicitly deal with conceptions of persons and respect for persons. The main focus for the nurse is interacting with persons within a health care environment and the term person is an evaluative moral term not a natural term used to describe objects or things in the world.

Teichman (1985) remarks that an attempted analysis of the concept of the person cannot be taken for granted in that it will, to some extent, be guided by ordinary use. The same may be said about the concept of care. In identifying features related to a concept of the person and the concept of care, it seems to be the case that variation in meaning and use will exist and highly individualistic viewpoints emerge. To some extent this may be because the concept of care, like the concept of the person, does not have a formal definition and it is, therefore, difficult to ground in any formal foundational knowledge. However, it may be possible to ground both concepts in commonsense knowledge. The moral features of both concepts could be supported by knowledge from the ethical domain. The learning experience obviously may influence how we construe things, persons and care and there may be a strong argument for teaching, through the ethical curriculum, the conceptions of the nature of care and the conceptions of persons. (Read Chapter 16, A study paper.)

Persons, non-persons and rights

It is claimed by some philosophers that, not only should rights be meaningfully predicated to persons but that it is conceptually possible and ethically correct to predicate rights to other animals who may not have person status. The question arises, "Could we ascribe person status to them, too?" Nazi Germany stripped a whole ethnic group of their person status by denying their rights and treating them as sub-human (see Dennett's themes, e.g. reciprocity, attitude and stance – the social influence of the concept of persons).

Some animals are close to being classified as a person, e.g. the chimpanzee. Why do we not ascribe person status to chimpanzees? Is it because they belong to another 'form of life' (Wittgenstein – "If a lion could speak we would not understand him")(Henry, 1986). Midgley (1983) remarks that we have no right to diminish the inner lives of the rest of creation and she defends the inner lives of non-language-using animals. An assessment of whether non-language using animals have a special kind of self-reflected consciousness of themselves may come from our own understanding within our own forms of life. Midgley remarks that we may give creatures of our own kind a preference in that it is a virtue to look after your own kind. She points out that the reason why animals matter is, in part, because they matter to themselves. She attributes notions of self- reflection and self-determination to non-language-using animals and this reflects an ability to be rational. Obviously, rational language-using animals (persons) could be included in her claim. We actually create in our phenomenological world (interpretive) our own concept of the person. We can understand our pet dog, communicate with him/her and may also personify and attribute human psychological terms to him or her.

If we ascribe person status and rights by social and ethical procedures, then, in turn, it is possible to ascribe person status to other beings besides humans.

SUMMARY OF KEY POINTS

i)   There are different ways of understanding the concept of the person. It is not perfectly rational or clear cut and it is difficult to define

ii) There are alternative ways of understanding (not defining) what is meant by the term person:

   a)   the term may be viewed as normative and a moral term, like the term good

b)   a person may be viewed as having special features

c)   in commonsense terms, the meaning of giving person status may depend upon how we use it in language and in context

iii)   The term person stands for what humans essentially are, and nurses and doctors professionally care for human persons

iv)   There are no clear dividing lines between persons and non-persons and it is the borderline cases that cause the problems

v)   A concept of care is linked closely to the concept of the person. The two concepts in this sense are not natural terms but can be viewed as moral terms because they do not describe objects or things

vi)   Both commonsense and ethical knowledge underpin the nurse's understanding of the concept of the person

DISCUSSION QUESTIONS

1. Discuss why someone may argue that:

    a) The foetus may not be a person because it lacks particular person features.

    b) This sort of viewpoint on defining persons will not work.

2. Can the severely mentally handicapped individual be a person or not?

3. Why may it be necessary for the nurse practitioner to know about the term person being an undefinable concept?

4. What particular perspectives should we take when caring for persons: the moral, the feature list, or meaning in commonsense terms, or all three?

5. Is it possible to ascribe person status to the non-human?

6. Why is the concept 'care' (specifically health care) linked to the concept of person?

Chapter 6
Autonomy and paternalism

AUTONOMY

Being an autonomous person demands moral respect (see Chapter 5). Persons have the ability to govern their own conduct by rules and values, having freedom of choice and taking responsibility for their actions. Respecting a person as being autonomous means also respecting persons as ends in themselves (see Chapter 8, under Kantian ethics, p48). In other words, persons are autonomous to the extent to which they are able to control their own lives and their own destiny, using their own faculties. Persons are not passive but active beings (Henry, 1987). However, full autonomy is an ideal notion and we can only approximate to it. It is obvious that, in reality, some situations, states and circumstances will diminish a person's autonomy (such as, the ability to control his or her desires or actions, or both) through being restricted in some way, e.g. illness, psychological impairment, physical or mental disability.

Autonomy is part of the value of life. There is no such thing as complete autonomy, only maximal autonomy. This involves a person being reasonably autonomous in all circumstances.

> *Consider:*   *no apparent defect in control.*
> *no apparent defect in reasoning.*
> *no apparent defect in information.*

PATERNALISM

The definition of paternalism involves the belief that it can be right to order the lives of others for their own good, irrespective of their wishes or judgements.

Paternalism may only be justified for so long as it takes to appraise the person of the defects in his or her decisions.

The only thing that makes paternalism morally respectable is its claim to be an essential part of a respect for persons. However, paternalist concerns for the welfare of others cannot be consistent with respect for them as persons where the agents choices are maximally autonomous (Harris, 1985).

Basically, paternalism holds that health professionals should take a parental role towards patients and their families. Professionals have superior knowledge of medicine; they alone have a right to decide what is best for patients and their families because of their long and specialised training. The medical and nursing profession may support this by the following arguments:

1. Lay people lack professional knowledge of medicine in dealing with physical/mental illness or injury and therefore, have no way of knowing what is best for them.

2. Through a long hard period of professional education and their experiences, professionals, especially doctors, know the characteristics of diseases and injury. Therefore, patients should place themselves totally in the professionals' hands.

3. Any or all decisions about patients care and treatment, including the information that should be given to them, should be in the hands of doctors and their professional assistants.

However, this is not necessarily consistent with health care in that it is said that patients have rights over their own bodies and lives. Respect for a person's autonomy is central. Further, doctors are human persons capable of error too. Often decisions involve not just medical concerns and doctors are not qualified to make decisions about these. Finally, paternalism often leads to total patient dependence on doctors and sometimes results in dehumanisation (Thiroux, 1977).

SUMMARY OF KEY POINTS

Autonomy

i) To be autonomous means we are able to control our own lives and to some extent our destiny. It means having freedom of choice and taking responsibility

ii) Full autonomy is an ideal notion and we can only approximate to it

iii) A person's autonomy may be diminished through circumstances or situations, e.g. illness

Paternalism

i) Paternalism is a belief that it can be right to order the lives of others for their own good

ii) Paternalism is morally respectable only in its claim to be essential for respect for persons

iii) Respect for persons is central and paternalism can lead to total patient dependence, i.e. loss of autonomy

DISCUSSION QUESTIONS

1. Who should make judgements about a person's defect in autonomy? The doctor, the nurse, both or none? Discuss.

2. Can we view autonomy as an absolute for persons in the health care field?

3. Should the patient be viewed as passive or active?

4. What is paternalism and why is it so much a part of health care?

5. Is there any situation within health care in which one can justify paternalism? Discuss.

6. Why should the nurse practitioner need to understand these two terms, autonomy and paternalism?

Chapter 7
Rights

According to Hospers (1973), a 'right' is a moral principle defining and sanctioning a person's freedom of action in a social context.
One explanation for rights is where a social rule gives the individual rights. However, underlying the social rule is the moral notion, i.e. "one ought to have that right."
To examine some of the problems that one may encounter over arguments for rights involves looking at a claim for insisting upon absolute rights.
Absolute rights bring to the fore the notion of natural rights. A person, it is said, has an absolute right, naturally by being human. The misconception is that a right as such, is not a property of the person, like an arm or a leg or the capacity to think and feel. (A right is not like a descriptive fact or thing.)
It may be claimed that a woman has an absolute right over her own body, including procreative rights. Women have claimed that because of the accident of nature, they get pregnant and therefore, in the past, have not shared equal rights with men. Birth control now gives them the opportunity for equal rights. Further, abortion from this point of view is seen as a form of birth control. Their argument develops where the foetus is seen as part of a woman's body, at least until it is born. Therefore, she has an absolute right over whether it should or shouldn't continue to live in that body.
The problem in this case is not just that the foetus is misrepresented as being only a simple organ of the woman's body, but the claim made for absolute rights. Conflicting claims cannot

35

be solved, e.g. the woman's right over her own body and the man's right to protection of his potential child. It is also possible that we endow some rights to the later developing foetus (see Persons, Henry 1986).

Rights involve 'other regarding' situations for other people and for the protection and value we place on the person. They involve someone in a social relationship with the person upon whom those duties rest. This applies to the professional rights of the nurse and the moral rights of the patient. One question that can be raised in relation to the pregnant woman's situation is, "Does the potential mother have a relationship of any sort with the foetus she carries?" With the foetus's later development perhaps she does, both psychologically and physically. She sustains its life and psychologically responds to the sensory movements of the foetus. Further, if the foetus is denied rights as a human being or a separate person, then good reasons have to be given on moral grounds for denying those rights. If no relevant differences obtain between mother and the foetus then in no way can we deny those rights. The early foetus is very different but at the later stages the foetus is very much 'person-like' even though perhaps not a person in the full sense (see Chapter 5, Persons).

In the case of the nurse who cares for the patient, she too has a duty to uphold the rights of the patient, particularly to treatment and nursing care. The nurse's views regarding abortion may, in fact, conflict with the woman who claims an absolute right over her body and consents to abortion. If we take the notion that absolute rights cannot obtain in a social situation but rights must still take high priority, the nurse has the right to withhold her involvement in the abortion procedure but not the right to stop 'caring' for the patient.

She must uphold her duty to the patient's right to nursing care procedures. The right to professional care is 'other regarding' and both social and ethical. The claim for an abortion based upon the notion of an absolute right is not ethically sound and usually other factors are taken into consideration before an abortion is carried out. ('Absolute right to life' claims by the anti-abortionists also run into difficulties.)

To define rights as an individual's power to control action and forbearance of others is not justified. If this was the case it would simply mean that adults in society in a contractual fashion would exercise those rights. The very young child or the mentally handicapped would have no rights, simply because they could not exercise them. Underlying any law or social rule giving rights is the value we place upon the person. Children, the mentally handicapped, the old and infirm all have rights protected by others. (The person is valued.) Unfortunately, human rights are not recognised in all societies; certainly not in some third world countries. In this sense we must not presume that rights are universal.

The important point about rights is that a generality of moral obligation lays down the general terms by which one can accept the notion of human rights. The rights of the mentally handicapped can be protected by others on moral grounds. Rights are prescriptive in that they are indicative of moral obligation. The notion of natural rights implies that by being human there is an indication of having rights of some kind. The term 'human' must not be taken to mean just species membership; it also implies personhood. Further, we impose rights and duties on other non-persons, especially if they are like us, e.g. we speak of animal rights. And the foetus at a later state is not only a member of our species but is strikingly like us.

Imposing rights on non-persons involves a psychological feature of persons. Indirectly, there is a psychological element when we also speak of natural rights in terms of our own moral standards.

Typically, rights have been seen as being possessed or owned by individuals. However, it is the **notion** behind the right that entails having moral justification.

A right-based theory is founded upon what is good for people or in their interests. A right-based theory will foster tolerance and liberty. Underpinning this is respect for the dignity and autonomy of persons that is an 'end in ourselves' (Benjamin Curtis, 1981).

SUMMARY OF KEY POINTS

i) Moral rights are viewed as expressing moral principles

ii) Rights sanction a person's freedom of action in a social context

iii) A right is not like a descriptive fact; it is prescriptive

iv) With absolute rights conflicting claims cannot be solved

v) The patient's rights involve the nurse upholding her duty to patients

vi) Underlying any law or social rule that gives the person rights is respect for persons

vii) Human rights are not recognised in all societies so rights are not universal

viii) A right fosters liberty, respect, dignity and autonomy of persons

DISCUSSION QUESTIONS

1. Can you have an absolute right? Discuss.

2. What happens when there is a conflict of rights?

3. Discuss why rights are not descriptive but prescriptive.

4. Can there be such a thing as 'animal rights'?

5. Why would the nurse practitioner have a duty to uphold the rights of the patient?

6. Why is it that some societies do not recognise 'human rights'?

counsey — ULTRI
TEOLOGICAL   EGO

Deological — ACT
ROLE.

Chapter 8
Two major perspectives of morality (teological and deontological)

CONSEQUENTIALIST APPROACH (TEOLOGICAL)

In the history of ethics, two major viewpoints emerge traditionally known as the teological and deontological theories respectively. The two major consequentialist theories are egoism and 'utilitarianism, and both are based upon, or are concerned with, consequences. They differ in that they disagree on who should benefit from these consequences. The egoists say persons ought to act in their own self-interest, whereas utilitarians say that persons ought to act in the interests of all concerned and, therefore, a utilitarian view may be more useful in health care because of the 'other regarding' factor.

Ethical egoism

To clarify the situation it may be helpful to examine the differences between psychological egoism and ethical egoism. Psychological egoism is scientific and descriptive whereas ethical egoism is the normative prescriptive approach. The strong form of psychological egoism maintains that people will always act in their own self-interest and that they are psychologically constructed to do so, whereas the weak form states that persons often but not always act in their own self-interest. These two approaches cannot act as a basis for ethical egoism. Why tell people to do what they cannot help doing? With respect to the weak sense, if I often act

41

in my own self-interest, this has nothing to do with what I should or **ought** do.

Ethical egoism generally takes three forms:

1. Universal ethical egoism states the basic principle that I *should* act in my self-interest regardless of the interests of others unless those interests also serve me.

2. Individual ethical egoism states that everyone ought to act in 'my self-interest'.

3. Personal ethical egoism states that I ought to act in my own self-interest but that I make no claims about what anyone else ought to do.

There are obvious problems with points 2 and 3 in that they only apply to one individual and cannot be laid down for humanity in general. Universal ethical egoism is the most common version presented by egoists and represents a strong reaction to the ethics of traditional rules.

However, ethical egoism is self-contradictory in that it cannot be to one individual's advantage that others should pursue their own advantage. Further, an important part of morality is advising and judging and it seems ridiculous if A comes to B for moral advice and B advises A to do something by considering what is in B's own interests. Ethical egoism obviously is severely limited, particularly for the health care domain. The theory only works if it is used when people are in relative isolation, thereby minimising the conflicts.

Utilitarianism

The essence of utilitarianism lies in the effects which an action may be presumed to have and the fundamental point emphasised is the **consequences**, not motives of the agent.

The principal architects of utilitarianism were J. Bentham (1748–1832) and John Stewart Mills (1806–1873). Bentham maintained that what is good is pleasure or happiness and what is bad is pain. Therefore, one state of affairs is better than another if it increases the balance of pleasure over pain. Bentham devised a **hedonistic calculus** on a seven-point scale to measure the amount of pleasure over pain. However, Mills said that one could not quantify pleasures. He took over the **Principle of Utility** to try to articulate it but started from the same basis: 'everyone pursues pleasure'.

Act utilitarianism

Early utilitarianism was an attempt to lay down an objective principle for determining when a given action was right or wrong, the maxim being called the Principle of Utility. It was considered objectively right because it referred to an act as good in so far as it produces the greatest happiness for the greatest number. The essence of the utilitarian philosophy thus lies in the effects which an action may be presumed to have.

Rule utilitarianism

This is where the rightness or wrongness of an act is modified to the adoption of a rule and the calculation of the likely consequences of that rule under which the particular act falls. For example, a person known to be innocent, should never be found guilty.

In objection to the thesis of ethical relativism (see Chapter 4, Absolute and relative views) the rule utilitarian would state that there is at least one moral principle which should operate in all societies, that of rule utilitarianism. It applies to the rules, not to the moral principle from which the rules derive.

Basic problems with utilitarianism

"If every man always pursues his own pleasure, how
are we to secure that the legislator shall pursue the
pleasure of mankind in general'" (Russell 1974)

Kant urged that **you ought** implies **you can.** Conversely, if you
cannot, it is futile to say **you ought.** According to Kant if each man
must always pursue his own pleasure, ethics is reduced to
prudence.

One difficulty with utilitarianism is that it assumes that the
total number of effects must be taken into account before an
action can be assessed as right or wrong. If we merely count the
immediate amount of pleasure and pain we may be mistaken,
since the long-range effects may give different results. Therefore,
if we can never assess the rightness or wrongness of an act until we
know all of its effects, we shall have to wait indefinitely before
declaring the act to be right or wrong because there may be an
infinite number of effects.

The utilitarians counter this criticism by saying that we can
determine the rightness or wrongness of an action with a high
degree of probability without waiting for all the consequences to
happen. However, this depends too strongly on subjectivism and
speculation, e.g. a man's belief that the act in question is likely to
have desirable consequences. Further, rule utilitarianism seems to
necessitate careful qualification of each rule. When can we find
the best rule?

The positive aspect of utilitarianism is the notion that
intention and a sense of duty are not the sole criteria of moral
worth. However, can our acts be properly evaluated without some
consideration of the motives from which they are done? Examples
are gratitude (perhaps to parents) which is not based on any
probable future consequences, and justice, e.g. equal treatment or
treatment in accord with dessert.

SUMMARY OF KEY POINTS

Ethical egoism

i) Ethical egoism is a normative prescriptive theory and universal ethical egoism is the most commonly held version

ii) Ethical egoism will only work as long as people are in relative isolation from each other, thereby minimising conflicts

iii) We do not live in isolated communities and we need other ethical theories

Utilitarianism

i) Utilitarianism maintains that everyone should perform that act or follow that moral rule which will bring about the greatest good or happiness for everyone

ii) Act utilitarianism states that everyone should perform that act which will bring about the greatest good over bad. The act utilitarian believes that one cannot establish rules in advance to cover all situations because they are all different

iii) Rule utilitarianism states that everyone should always follow the rules which will bring about the greatest number of good consequences for all. However, it is not only difficult to determine what would be good consequences, it is difficult to be sure that a rule can be established to cover the diversity of human motives and actions

iv) The consequentialist theories demand that we discover and determine all the consequences of our actions or rules. This is virtually impossible to achieve

DISCUSSION QUESTIONS

1. Why is the utilitarian theory considered an objective theory?

2. Why would ethical egoism be even more limited within the health care domain?

3. What is the difference between these two consequential theories?

4. Discuss how the utilitarian theory might be useful within the health care system.

NON-CONSEQUENTIALIST APPROACH (DEONTOLOGICAL)

Non-consequential theories fall into two categories, act and rule, like consequentialist theories, the main difference being that the non-consequential theories are not based upon consequences.

ACT NON-CONSEQUENTIALISTS

Act non-consequentialists state that there are no general moral rules or theories at all, only particular actions, situations and people about which we cannot generalise. Each situation must be approached individually and it is now we decide which is more important. This theory is sometimes known as the intuitionist approach.

The theory is characterised by "If it feels good, do it." Traditionally, it is like the emotive and non-cognitive theories of morality. The emotive theory, for instance, states that ethical words and sentences do two things:

i)   Express people's feelings and attitudes
ii)   evoke certain feelings and attitudes of others.

Reasons for accepting intuition are:

i)   Any well-meaning person has a sense of right and wrong
ii)   Human beings had moral ideas and convictions long before philosophers created ethics
iii)   Reasoning on moral matters will confirm our intuitions but our reasoning can go wrong and therefore we must fall back on moral insights and intuitions

Reasons for rejecting intuition are:

i)   The word intuition has come to mean hunches that lack scientific and philosophical respectability

ii) It is difficult to define intuition and to prove its existence. There is no proof that we have an inborn or innate set of moral rules with which we might compare our acts to see whether they are moral or not

iii) Intuition is immune to objective criticism because it applies only to the possessor and one person's intuition may be different from another's

RULE NON-CONSEQUENTIALISTS

Rule non-consequentialists state that there are rules as a basis for morality and that consequences do not matter. The main way various rule non-consequentialists differ is in how they establish rules. The major rule non-consequentialist theory, sometimes known as duty ethics, was formulated by Immanuel Kant (1724 – 1804).

Kantian ethics

Kant was a rule deontologist and suggested only one basic principle. The key to answering questions such as "What is the nature of morality?" and "What is a moral action by contrast with a non-moral action?" lay in distinguishing between acts done from inclination and acts done from a sense of duty.

Inclination must also be distinguished from obligation. Kant rejects the idea of acting upon one's inclinations with moral matters. A man is acting morally only when he suppresses feelings and inclinations, and does what he is obliged to do, e.g 'doing one's duty'.

There is a difference also between actions which are in accord with duty and those done from duty. The former are not necessarily moral but the latter are, e.g. parents who care for their children out of fear of prosecution from the law or because they are fond of them, act in accord with duty. It is only moral if they have a special obligation to their children because they are their children.

The essence of morality is to be found in the motive from which the act is done (not the consequences). According to Kant, nothing can possibly be conceived in the world, or even out of it without qualification except good will, and, if we ask, "What is good will?", it is acting for the sake of duty, not simply in accordance with duty. He goes on to say that there is a distinction between prudential actions and moral actions. A man who repays a debt because of the fear of the legal consequences, acts from a sense of prudence, not out of duty. He reasoned that one ought always to behave as if one's course of action or conduct were to become a universal law. This is why lying cannot be accepted as moral under any circumstances at all. An imperative is a command and within the field of morals, Kant distinguishes two types:

The hypothetical imperative *is where qualifications are attached, for example, "work hard if you want to succeed." This is usually prudential and involves a means to an end.*
The categorical imperative *is not concerned with achieving an end or purpose but is for its own sake. It enjoins actions without any 'ifs' and without any regard for the effect such an action may have and lays down rules which, if followed, will ensure that the person is behaving morally.*

Kant believed that the distinguishing feature of human beings was reason and rationality applicable to morals. One characteristic of reason is universality. "The same for all men everywhere and in all circumstances, thus the basic requirement of all moral action." Moral choice is not an individual matter but an activity shared with other persons, all of whom equally with oneself, are ends in themselves.

Some basic problems with Kantian philosophy

Kant does not handle cases where we have a conflict of duties. If one promises to keep a secret and then someone asks you to tell the truth, one cannot keep a promise and at the same time tell the truth. Yet, according to Kant, you should do both. In such a situation we cannot logically universalise behaviour.

A person may be mistaken in his or her understanding of what constitutes duty. As a result the person might do something which is morally wrong.

It seems unnecessarily harsh to deny moral goodness to persons who, as a result of deliberate self-discipline and self-habituation, have so disposed themselves to kindliness that helping others comes to them like second nature, without inner conflict or any idea of doing their duty.

Finally, Kant seems to be urging too strong a claim when he insists that we should never tell lies. (This is universalising.) Moral rules should only be interpreted as generalisations rather than categorical propositions without expectations. There may be circumstances when one has to lie and may be obligated morally to do so. Telling the truth and keeping promises are obligations which one should keep, providing no overriding factors are present.

SUMMARY OF KEY POINTS

i)   Act non-consequentialist theories do not concern rules: intuitionism is based upon what people feel (intuit) is right or wrong

ii)   Rule non-consequentialist theories claim that there are rules which are the basis of morality and consequences do not matter. The rules are moral commands which are right

iii) Kantian rules are universalised

iv) The Kantian golden rule is: "Would you want this done to you?"

v) Kant emphasised duties over inclinations and gave no rule for what we should do when our inclinations and duties are the same

DISCUSSION QUESTIONS

1. Intuition focuses on the questionable assumption that all situations and people are completely different and they have nothing in common. Is that true?

2. How can a nurse practitioner resolve conflict of duty?

3. Are there some rules that may be universalised yet not necessarily be moral?

4. Should there be some kind of synthesis between consequential and non-consequential theories?

5. Discuss the differences between act and rule non-consequentialist theories

Chapter 9
Informed consent and confidentiality

♥ INFORMED CONSENT

The term consent is ambiguous. Downie and Calman (1987) remark that it means granting someone permission to do something he/she would not have the right to do without such permission.

Gillon (1985) says it means a voluntary decision, made by a sufficiently competent or autonomous person on the basis of information and deliberation, to accept a proposed course of action. Consent in this sense requires action by an autonomous agent based on adequate information and refers to informed consent.

Informed consent involves respect for each others autonomy and therefore respect for persons.

Doing things without consent means ignoring a person's autonomy (person status, see Chapter 5, Persons).

An important point to bear in mind is that consent is a concept which relates not just to clinical trials and experimental research but to any relationship between patient or client and the health care professional.

Basic moral principles of health care involving consent must consider the following:

i)   Respect for a person's autonomy
ii)   Protection of patients and subjects involved in research
iii)   Avoidance of fraud, duress or anxiety
iv)   The use of self-audit by the professionals in order to scrutinise their own motives in wishing to suggest treatments or procedures
v)   Promotion of rational decisions by the professionals and the promotion of public social values

Consent can be viewed in three ways: a legal device designed to protect a person and autonomy; legal protection for the professional if things go wrong; or as an extension of patient–doctor, patient–professional relationships built upon trust (Downie *et al.* 1987).

To consent to medical intervention a person requires sufficient information to be able to make an informed and deliberated choice, and it is in this context that doctors often object. Patients may be unnecessarily alarmed and their medical state unnecessarily impaired if given information about the diagnosis or prognosis or risks associated with the proposed management of treatment. However, it is dangerous to extrapolate from the doctor's own position to generalisations about patients. Further there should be respect for the patient's autonomy, i.e. what and how much the patient wants to know (psychological understanding).

Consent in English law leaves the doctor to decide in the context of their therapeutic relationships, how much information they ought to give when obtaining consent for treatment. Nevertheless, laws do not in themselves, provide moral justification.

CONFIDENTIALITY

Confidentiality concerns rights, privacy, respect for a person's autonomy, and involves both deontological and utilitarian issues. Most codes of conduct hold that the rule of confidentiality is not absolute and ought to be viewed as a guide line for ethical reasoning. The problem surrounds how to interpret and apply confidentiality remembering confidentiality as a principle has its limits.

Confidentiality is:

i)   Based on the hippocratic oath as authority because the oath holds confidentiality as a universal principle

ii)   A belief that professionals will keep confidences and this enables the patient to seek help without stigma or repercussions. Its utility is in keeping doctors in work, encouraging patients to seek help and preserving a healthy society. This may encourage mutual trust which is important for the patient/doctor relationship

iii)   An expressed or an implied contract between professional and patient built upon the understanding that information will be kept secret (a commonsense knowledge)

iv)   Personal control over information about oneself is important. Access to such information relates to love, friendship and trust. For a utilitarian justification privacy is useful and would be lost without reasonable expectation that health care professionals should or ought to keep confidences. The deontological issues could relate to a duty the professional has to maintain privacy and respect the person as autonomous

SUMMARY OF KEY POINTS

Informed consent

i)   Consent requires action by an autonomous agent

ii)   Consent involves respect for persons

iii) Consent protects a person's autonomy, the professional and involves a relationship of trust between patient and doctor

Confidentiality

i)   Confidentiality is not absolute but provides a guideline for ethical reasoning

ii)   It involves rights, privacy, autonomy and deontological and utility issues

DISCUSSION QUESTIONS

1.   What is really meant by informed consent; can the lay person ever be fully informed?

2.   Why would informed consent be required in non-therapeutic research?

3.   How and to what extent is confidentiality a requirement of the health care professional's respect for his or her patients or clients?

4.   What sort of reasons for treating confidentiality as absolute will resort in harm or suffering to others?

5.   Should the nurse practitioner be prepared to defend breaking of confidentiality or not?

Chapter 10
Reproductive technology and embryonic research

REPRODUCTIVE TECHNOLOGY

Decisions regarding infertility centre upon the Warnock Report (1985).

ARTIFICIAL INSEMINATION

This procedure involves concentrated semen being inserted into the uterus of the female partner (if the male is not completely infertile). The only arguments against this are that it separates the initiative and procreative functions of sexual intercourse and it involves the male partner masturbating, which some consider wrong.

N.P However, having a male donor is more controversial because the semen comes from a donor who is not the male partner. A third party is introduced into the relationship and the effect on the potential child may cause problems. Nevertheless, the practice is carried out in a clinical setting, the identity of the donor is secret, consent is given and no sexual intercourse is involved.

N.P. If one considers the consequences on the child, empirical considerations are important. In support of the procedure, the partners are consulted and counselled. A childless partnership may not be good for both partners and the psychological and social issues must be taken into account.

The law in Britain is problematic although the Warnock Report does recommend the law be altered so that couples adopt a child conceived in this way. However, if the potential child wishes to know the identity of the genetic father, disclosure of such information may have an adverse effect on the recruitment of donors. Perhaps it is worth mentioning briefly that these arguments can be extended to surrogacy. However, the Warnock report disapproves because of the possibility of commercial exploitation (see the Warnock Report, 1985).

N.P. in *vitro* **fertilisation** is a relatively new development and is useful for five percent of infertile couples. Through the process of in *vitro* fertilisation (IVF), the ripe egg is extracted from the ovary, mixed with semen and then transferred to the uterus of the carrying mother. There is some difficulty regarding implantation and, for this reason, several eggs must be harvested and fertilised. The production of more eggs is achieved by artificial stimulation of the woman's ovaries so that several eggs are produced in one cycle.

This process of IVF can be used in a number of ways: husband and wife may both be donors and re-implantation is into the wife's uterus; or donor sperm and the wife's egg may be re-implanted into the wife's uterus; or donor sperm or husband's sperm and the wife's egg may be re-implanted in a female third party (surrogacy). All these raise different moral issues but two arguments are often used against IVF.

First, the practice is seen as unnatural; however, in one sense medical intervention itself can be viewed as unnatural and, therefore, the unnatural claim does not hold. The two terms natural and unnatural are really rhetoric, not argument. Secondly, concerns are raised for resources for research priorities. This is viewed as a stronger argument against prioritising resources for IVF over and above other areas of medical care and life saving services.

Obviously, technical and moral problems arise over difficulties of re-implantation. To minimise the difficulties in practice, several embryos are transferred to the potential mother in order to increase the chance of pregnancy. Two moral problems arise. First, the possibility of multiple pregnancy, which may result in risks to the mother, and secondly, the fate of surplus embryos.

EMBRYONIC RESEARCH

The first two months after conception is known as the embryonic period. After the second month, the developing human is known as the foetus. Immediately after fertilisation there is rapid division and by the third day there are sixteen cells. Usually around the fourth or fifth day the cluster of cells, know as a blastocyst, is like a hollow ball. The outer layer of cells will form the placenta and the inner layer of cells and the fluid-filled space will produce the developing embryo. It is usually at seven to eight days that implantation occurs and the blastocyst is no more than one-hundredth of an inch in diameter. At twelve days further rapid changes occur and usually around the fourteenth day there are signs of the primitive streak being formed. It is not until forty days have elapsed that there are signs of a rudimentary brain, spinal cord and upper and lower extremities.

The **Embryonic Bill** will become law for the regulation and limiting of research on human embryos up to fourteen days old. However, behind every law there should be a moral maxim. Political debate ought to take into account all moral issues underpinning legislation. A Statutory Licensing Authority will monitor the embryonic research.

The question arises of what to do with the left over embryos created in *vitro*. For instance, is it morally acceptable to allow them to die or use them for research?

A central moral principle of health care and research is respect for persons as autonomous individuals (Downie and Calman, 1987). However, for many people, particularly in relation to embryonic research, the moral issues surround the question of when does life begin? For most people the answer to that question determines when respect ought to be shown. Some people will say that life begins at conception and therefore insist that abortion and embryonic research is morally wrong. We can take the obvious notion that embryonic research involves experimentation on a potential human being or a potential person.

In a biological sense it is simply not true that life begins at conception. Life is constantly evolving and conception is only one stage. The sperm and the unfertilised ovum are both alive and this line of thinking leads us into a reductionistic argument. The question of when does life begin is difficult to answer so the question must be changed. The question asked could be: at what stage of development should the status of person be accorded to the human embryo? However, once again some will say at fertilisation; others at implantation and so on. The question is also not a question of fact but of decision and judgement and no answer is possible.

Warnock remarks that the special status of the human embryo and its protection by law does not depend upon when it becomes a person. This is simply because first, we cannot give an answer to the question of when or at what stage of development the developing human becomes a person and secondly, if full person status is given to the early embryo, then such status demands the rights and legal enactments properly accorded to full persons.

Unfortunately, it is not clear what special status the embryo is given by the recommendations of the Warnock report and this is often one of the major criticisms levelled at the Warnock Committee. The only reference to the status of the embryo is the idea that the embryo demands more status than other animal subjects. However, other animal subjects used in experimentation have no status or rights at all.

A discussion on the claim for giving special status to the embryo, i.e. that of potential personhood, will also lead us into difficulties. However, if the embryo has special status because it is a potential person then legal protection of its development must be adhered to. Unfortunately, it does not follow that, because an embryo has potential to become a person, it should be allowed or assisted to become a person. The sperm and unfertilised egg also have this potential. We cannot be viewed as having a duty to fertilise every unfertilised egg. However, it may be argued that after fertilisation, the potential becomes stronger. Further, it does not follow from the fact that if something is a potential person, we should treat it as a person, i.e. that it should have the same rights and respect. We are all potentially dead, but that is not to say that we should be treated as such. Nevertheless, although the potential argument is not sufficient, further clarification on what we mean and how we use the term 'potential' should be followed through.

The question raised should perhaps be changed again into: at what stage does the developing human have moral significance? Or, how much moral significance does the embryo have?

According to Warnock, the embryo is not a person and may be viewed as a collection of cells. It is only at implantation that the embryo has potential. However, Hare (1987) claims that we should take account of the potential person into whom an embryo might grow, if implanted, or the potential people that might be brought into being if other embryos were implanted. Hare (1987) remarks that the Warnock Committee does not give good reasons for allowing experimentation up to fourteen days and there should be an examination of the consequences for all those affected. In other words we should enquire into the good and harm that would come from allowing or forbidding embryonic research.

The Warnock report suggests that experiments should be carried out only by properly licensed bodies and only during the first fourteen days. The moral significance given to the developing human becomes more important with the development of the brain and CNS which creates the possibility of pain and sensory cognition. Feeling pain and the development of cognition are both features that are attributed to persons (see Henry, 1986). Further, Warnock remarks that viability and individuality is another important stage in the acquisition of moral rights. On the one hand Warnock is correct in claiming that the embryo is not a person, although potentiality for becoming a person cannot be ruled out. However, Warnock discusses the potentiality argument as not being appropriate for affording special status to the embryo. Nevertheless, the reasons for the special status accorded to the embryo by Warnock are not clear.

If the embryo has no special status then it cannot be given absolute respect or rights. The embryo has no legal status or right to life.

The Warnock report recommends limiting research on embryos. The embryo must not be used for research beyond fourteen days and, if used within fourteen days, never transferred to a woman. Further, it is essential to obtain informed consent from the donors of spare embryos. The question arises: what is informed consent?

SUMMARY OF KEY POINTS

Reproductive technology: Artificial insemination and in *vitro* fertilisation

i) Artificial insemination involves concentrated semen being inserted into the uterus of a female partner

ii) The consequences to the potential child involve empirical considerations and the law in Britain is problematic in relation to adoption

iii) In support of the procedure partners are consulted and counselled

61

iv) Ripe eggs are harvested from the ovary, mixed with semen and then re-implanted in the uterus in the process called in *vitro* fertilisation

v) Artificial insemination and in *vitro* fertilisation are both viewed as unnatural processes

vi) Resources for IVF are needed but are balanced against other priorities for medical care

Embryonic research

i) The embryonic stage is known as the first two months after fertilisation

ii) The embryonic bill will become law for the regulation and limiting of research on human embryos up to fourteen days

iii) Many people, particularly in relation to embryonic research, will ask the question: when does life begin? The answer to that question determines when respect ought to be shown

iv) The question can be changed to: at what stage of development should the status of a person be accorded? This question is not a question of fact but of decision and judgement and no answer is possible

v) It is not clear what special status, if any, is given to the embryo

vi) There are difficulties with using the 'potential-person' argument for giving the embryo special status even if it cannot be given person status

vii) Informed consent must be obtained from potential parents. What is meant by informed consent?

viii) Consequences should be considered when enquiring into the good and harm that would come from allowing or forbidding embryonic research

DISCUSSION QUESTIONS

1. Is the practice of using a donor for artificial insemination wrong in itself or because of the consequences for the potential child?

2. Would your attitude towards artificial insemination alter if the couple were not married or homosexual/lesbian?

3. Should information about the donor remain confidential?

4. What importance do you attach to the findings of research into reproductive technology as opposed to cancer research?

5. When does life begin?

6. Discuss when you think life may have moral significance.

7. Does the embryo have special status or not? Discuss.

8. Discuss the advantages and disadvantages of legalising embryonic research.

Chapter 11
Some issues on euthanasia

The word euthanasia comes from the Greek and originally meant 'a good and happy death'. In the 20th century it was interpreted as **mercy killing**. Mercy killing in most countries is legally seen as a form of murder.

The distinction between **active** and **passive** euthanasia is thought to be crucial for medical ethics (Rachels, 1975). The idea is that it is permissible, at least in some cases, to withhold treatment and allow a patient to die, but never to take any direct action designed to kill a patient.

Allowing someone to die implies that there is some point in any terminal illness when further curative treatment has no purpose. A patient in this situation should be allowed to die a natural death in comfort, peace and dignity. It does not involve active termination of a person's life. It involves a refusal to start curative treatment but does not mean that the patient should be abandoned to die in pain and misery. (This links to hospice care and it refers to dignity and respect for persons.)

According to Thiroux (1980), **mercy death** means taking direct action to terminate a person's life because the person has requested it (assisted suicide). Thiroux takes his own position in deciding not to use the term euthanasia to stand for both allowing someone to die and mercy killing because it blurs the distinction between acts of murder and what is merely good medical practice, i.e. allowing people to die of natural causes. Mercy killing refers to someone taking a direct action to terminate a person's life without the person's permission. The decision to take such an action is often made on the assumption that the person's life is no longer meaningful or that if the person was able to say so, he or she would express a desire to die. This involves assessment by others of the quality of life and what constitutes death (see Chapter 12, Transplants).

So far, allowing someone to die a natural death is legally sanctioned, whereas mercy death (voluntary) and mercy killing (involuntary) are not legal in this country. All three can be seen to relate to passive and active euthanasia. It is perhaps important to raise issues relating to the conception of death, in particular brain death, simply because they relate to decisions on the quality of life and withdrawal of medical support and treatment. Further confusion arises between brain death and allowing someone to die.

Technology allows for heart and lung functioning even if the person has irreversible brain damage or brain death (often important for transplants, see Chapter 12). The activity of the person is reduced to a biological organism with a beating heart and breathing lungs. An *ad hoc* committee at Harvard Medical School (1968) decided on criteria for determining brain death (see Chapter 12).

Persons can be declared medically dead even though their heart and lungs are still functioning. If a person is declared dead in the medical sense, no illegal act has been committed. (In lay-man terms this concerns perceptions of an expert's authority, and experience). However, many people confuse brain death with allowing someone to die or mercy killing by disconnecting the machine. Mercy killing or allowing someone to die may occur when the brain is severely damaged but does not meet the criteria for brain death; then quality of life assessments are involved and this raises controversial issues for the medical and health care team.

SUMMARY OF KEY POINTS

i)   Euthanasia originally means a good and happy death

ii)   Distinctions between active and passive euthanasia are thought to be crucial

iii)   Allowing someone to die does not mean that patients should be in pain and misery; rather that dignity and respect for persons must be accorded to them

iv)   Mercy death means taking direct action to terminate someone's life with their permission

v)   Mercy killing means taking direct action to terminate someone's life without their permission

DISCUSSION QUESTIONS

1.   What is the difference between active and passive euthanasia?

2.   What is the difference between mercy death and mercy killing?

3.   What is permissible in this country?

4.   Discuss why confusion may arise between withdrawal of medical support because of brain death and allowing someone to die.

Chapter 12
Transplants

Defining when life begins and when life ends is important for consideration of brain death and the use of organs for transplantation.

Defining death

Making the diagnosis of brain death and switching off the ventilator raises many moral questions.

The concept of **brain death** emerged in France in 1959. A group of French neurosurgeons described a condition which they termed death of the central nervous system. By the late 1960s the increasing number of organ transplantations and greater successes in technological care provided a background of the need for greater philosophical clarity concerning what it meant to be dead. Lack of such clarity was reflected in the ambiguous and often confusing terminology used at that time. The construct brain death achieved a degree of precision and was popular.

The Havard criteria for brain death are:

1. Absence of cerebral responsiveness
2. Absence of induced or spontaneous movement
3. Absence of spontaneous respiration
4. Absence of brainstem and deep tendon reflexes

EEG was deemed to be of great confirmatory value but performance of an EEG was not mandatory.

Two conditions mimic brain death: hypothermia and drug intoxication; therefore, tests should be repeated over 24 hours. Since the introduction of the Harvard criteria, numerous patients throughout the world have been diagnosed as brain dead, maintained on ventilators and observed until their heart stopped. No patient meeting the Harvard criteria has ever recovered.

In the years that followed publication of the Harvard report, it was gradually realised that a clinically testable component of brain death was death of the brain stem. In its upper part the brainstem contains crucial centres responsible for generating the capacity for consciousness, whereas in its lower part it contains the respiratory centre. (It is worth remembering the controversy in defining consciousness in pure physiological terms (see Valentine, 1982).) Signs and symptoms of brain stem death are apnoic coma with absent brain stem reflexes. Traditional views of death are not necessarily defined in these physiological terms. However, in medical terms it becomes a necessary and sufficient condition of death.

Brain stem death must not be confused with massive brain damage largely confined to the cerebral hemispheres, sparing much of the brain stem and the capacity to breath.

Some organs such as kidney and corneas do not need to be obtained from a donor whose heart is still beating, whereas others, such as heart, lung and liver do. Hence the criteria for death becomes pressing! The traditional definition of death, i.e. cessation of all cardiopulmonary activity, would exclude all heart, lung and liver transplants. Therefore, the traditional view of death must be overthrown to allow beating-heart donors to be classified as dead.

Organ transplantation qualifies as a life-and-death matter in two ways: first for the recipient, and, secondly, for the donor.

Transplants

Recipient's point of view

The fact that the person is taking a bodily organ from someone else does not appear to raise any ethical difficulty. However, one sort of case in which organ transplantation does seem morally objectionable from the recipient's point of view, is that in which an experimental procedure was carried out, not to benefit the recipient, but only to further medical science. (*Dr Bailey, California, 1984, transplanted the heart of a baboon into a child who died a week later: The Case of Baby Fae, Fitzpatrick, 1988.*)

Donor's point of view

A corpse is no longer a subject of a right in the strictest sense of the word for it is deprived of personality which alone can be a subject of a right (see Chapter 7, Rights). Death is seen as a necessary and sufficient condition of death of personality; that is, the person no longer exists in this world anyway!

If the person has given permission during their life-time then there should be no objection to a surgeon removing organs donated with consent. (Remember what is meant by informed consent.)

Further, removing an organ from a corpse does not attack the basic good of a human person if there is no human person, only the remains.

Many people believe that brain death is a sufficient indication of the absence of human life or personhood, even if the body displays some residual powers. It is argued, however, whether personhood and brain functioning are related as closely as supporters claim. (Doctors totally agree, nurses more unsure, teachers even more unsure: Henry, 1986.)

If we admit that there is a psychosocial part of each person and that everything should not be reduced to the physiological realm, then questions may be asked relating to traditional criteria for death. This would lead to restricting transplantations of heart, lung and liver.

RESOURCE ALLOCATION

Not all transplantations can be objected to on the grounds of resource allocation, since kidney transplantation is more cost effective than renal dialysis.

SUMMARY OF KEY POINTS

i)   Brain death means death of the brain stem which contains crucial centres responsible for generating the capacity for consciousness

ii)   Brain stem death must not be confused with massive brain damage that may spare the brain stem

iii)   From the recipient's point of view, maintaining life is definitely to their benefit and taking a bodily organ from someone who has died does not necessarily seem morally objectionable

iv)   It is morally objectionable from the recipient's point of view if an experimental procedure was carried out only to benefit medical science

v)   From the donor's point of view, a corpse no longer has rights in the strictest sense of the word

vi)   Death is a necessary and sufficient condition for death of the personality

vii)   Consent for organ transplantation from the potential donor is essential

viii) Kidney transplantation is more cost effective than renal dialysis

DISCUSSION QUESTIONS

1. How do we tell that a person is dead?

2. Are you satisfied with the criteria of brain death?

3. What form of consent is necessary in relation to transplants?

4. What, if any, are the moral distinctions between the use of cornea, kidney, liver or heart and lung for the purposes of transplantation?

5. Can we justify keeping someone alive by providing him or her with organs from someone else?

6. Is it right in principle to remove organs from a dead body?

7. When do we decide a person is no longer a person?

8. Can there be mental activity in the total absence of any brain function?

9. Suppose one bed is vacant in a transplantation unit and two persons require the resource. Who should be treated, and should age, usefulness and moral character be considered? Discuss. (Example of possible recipients: A 70-year-old man living alone and a 40-year-old mother of four (one-parent family).)

10. Should research on transplants have priority over and above other life-saving techniques?

Chapter 13
Mentally handicapped and mentally ill

There are no particular ethical texts that deal specifically with the care and treatment of the mentally handicapped and mentally ill. Apply your ethical theory to the issues and read general text books and journal articles. It is useful to look at both legal and social policy issues, for example the policy for community care and institutional care.

The mature, rational adult is said to be self-determining and self-governing: attitudes, respect and rights are involved. When applied to the person who has a mental handicap there is obvious difficulty, some say, because the individual may not rationally understand

The inability to understand is a matter of degree and making judgements on levels of understanding should not perhaps rest with the professional alone. Attitudes held by professionals, who may take a paternalistic view, influence policy laid down within both community and institutional settings and lead to ethical issues.

The ethical issues underpinning care of the mentally handicapped and mentally ill involve a conception of person, ascribing personhood and the rights given to persons. It is an evaluative term that has moral status and relates to the central concern for respect for persons (see Chapter 5, Persons). Do we, for instance, view the senile elderly with psychiatric problems as not quite persons?

An important feature is that mentally handicapped individuals should not lack moral respect just because they lack the natural capacity to totally understand. Can we give personhood status dependent on the features a person has, such as rationality, the ability to reflect, the ability to communicate, or is it on moral grounds that we have to consider respect for persons and ascribed person status for the severely mentally handicapped? According to Fairburn (1988), being a person is about becoming responsible and would involve taking opportunities and exercising choices. However, we cannot totally rely upon this notion of being a person from having such abilities in the case of the mentally handicapped or mentally ill.

The moral notion of personhood involves dignity and respect and the severely mentally handicapped and mentally ill have to have respect and all the attending rights accorded to them on their behalf because they are members of a rational species (Teichman, 1985).

A causal model of understanding mental handicap is not appropriate because it incorporates the assumption that what people do, is not, despite appearances, freely chosen by them but governed by forces and factors over which they have no control, e.g. "He would marry young; he is from a broken home." This implies not rational thought on the agent's part but that underlying causal factors explain the action.

This raises the problem of a medical model for the care of the mentally handicapped. An alternative model of care is perhaps more appropriate. Those who do not fully embody the abilities of a fully autonomous adult (and this is not absolute because we are not perfectly rational or logical like sophisticated computers), such as babies, the mentally handicapped, severely mentally ill or comatosed patients, ought to be given respect and moral value. The rights and care accorded to them must be upheld for them on their behalf by the health care professional.

SUMMARY OF KEY POINTS

i) It is useful to look at legal and policy issues for care of the mentally ill or mentally handicapped, remembering that underpinning any law, legislation or policy there should be a moral maxim

ii) The inability to understand, for the mentally handicapped and mentally ill, is a matter of degree

iii) A paternalistic view may be taken in some cases, in relation to care

iv) Ethical issues involve conceptions of persons and views of personal autonomy when we accord respect to the mentally ill and mentally handicapped

v) The mentally handicapped or mentally ill should not lack moral respect just because they lack the ability to totally understand

vi) A causal medical model is not necessarily the appropriate model in which to view the mentally ill or mentally handicapped person

DISCUSSION QUESTIONS

1. Medical staff categorise the mentally ill and mentally handicapped. What ethical issues arise from using the medical model?

2. What rights should the severely mentally handicapped and mentally ill have?

3. What view of the person would be most appropriate in caring for the mentally ill or mentally handicapped?

Chapter 14
Justice and equality in health care

The concept of justice relates to equal distribution and equal opportunity in health care and is one virtue amongst many. Justice ought to be measured against other claims such as freedom or maximisation of happiness.

Justice refers to the part of morality devoted to the balance of claims and burdens amongst individuals in society and the features of justice include:

> Fairness and impartiality
> Rules to guide and follow
> Merit, desire and needs
> Equality and equity

The features of justice, particularly fairness and equality, are not considered good in themselves but the means of achieving certain ends.

The idea of **distributive** justice is concerned with comparative treatment of persons in similar conditions. In other words person must be treated alike, for example in emergency care or treatment.

According to Glover (1970) people should be treated equally except where there are some relevant differences between them, for example the mentally or physically handicapped. It may be considered unjust for equal treatment and care to be given when some people have greater needs.

If we relate distributive justice to dessert then indirectly it relates to **retributive justice**, for example if we give persons different rewards for making a larger or smaller contribution to the community. Further the mentally and physically handicapped cannot be rewarded less than others (see Chapter 13, Mentally handicapped and mentally ill).

Retributive justice relates to what people or society deserves. However, the question arises, "Who judges what is deserved?"

Magee (1978) summarises John Rawls' view of justice. Rawls puts forward two principles:

a) Everyone should have basic liberties
b) No difference in wealth should be tolerated unless the difference would be for the benefit of the poorest group in society

The first principle dominates the second principle.

Respect for persons is implicit in the first and second principles. Rawls also says we all would choose the second principle out of self interest, that is, putting a floor under our feet in case we were in a situation where we were disadvantaged.

Rawls' basic principle of justice is the notion of fairness in that people would agree to the second principle if they didn't know whether they were talented or stupid, rich or poor. He replaces the concept of **equality** with the concept of **equity** (fairness) (Warnock, 1977).

It is essential to bear in mind that the concepts of justice and fairness are not absolute virtues (see Chapter 4, Absolute and relative views).

Moral issues and principles lie behind the claim for equality of health care. However, the concept of equality is not an absolute value but a means to achieving an end. To pursue the good life we may call upon many values, for example freedom and equal opportunity. Any single concept which overrides all others will not necessarily solve the problems and conflicts that occur (competing claims for resources). The term equality is social, moral and prescriptive.

Warnock (1977) remarks that if we speak of natural rights, natural justice or laws, we are, in fact, speaking in terms of our own moral standards. If a political decision is made or taken (to form the NHS) then rights have been established. It is the prescriptive element that is important.

In society where social legislation occurs we need some kind of adjustment between conflicting claims and the idea of natural rights would make this impossible (see Chapter 7, Rights).

In one sense, a right to health care can only be given to an individual within a society where adjustment is made between conflicting claims. In third world countries whilst recognising the desirability of working towards the universal system (NHS) and equal opportunity for everyone for health care, the rate of progress must be governed by the relative claims of other ideas upon resources. Therefore, resources becomes an important issue and ideals of social justice include freedom from want, fairness and equality.

It is well recognised that there are differences in the level of care provided, both locally and on a national level. For example, historically, hospitals or special services grow around a particular local need or demand. In other instances special interests of doctors or other health care workers have established particular skills or treatment. They may relate to overt or covert political decisions to have a particular form of treatment available in limited places only, for example open heart surgery and transplant units. If this is justified in terms of utility then it raises questions of justice.

Two policies are currently discussed:

a)   More even distribution so that resources are reduced in one area and increased in another, or

b)   Resources moved from acute services to the community-based services, for example psychiatry and care of the mentally handicapped

Attempts are made to equalise the resources (justice) and to establish priorities (utility). The argument is between justice versus utility.

There is a requirement to respect persons equally when working for health care. This follows from the requirement to respect autonomy in all people and from work establishing basic criteria for personhood. General moral principles are involved such as fairness and equal consideration.

If persons are not respected equally, perhaps because of scarce resources, then discrimination by the society occurs. There is a price to pay dependent upon money rather than right. (This raises the question of whether human rights exist only in an ideal world.)

PRIVATE HEALTH CARE AND MEDICINE

Some health care and treatment is provided outside the NHS. There is a growing number of private nursing homes for the care of the elderly and an increase in the number of private hospitals and private health care insurance schemes. Doctors and nurses, if they choose, can undertake a certain amount of private consultancy or care. Further, other health professionals, particularly those allied to medicine such as the physotherapist, can quite easily work within the private sector. Moral discussion centres around issues such as longer waiting lists for non-critical care, due to consultants and health care teams working outside the NHS. The 'ability to pay' will disadvantage those on lower income and allow the higher income groups to bypass the NHS waiting list system. NHS resources may be used to enhance the private sector for example, laboratory and other NHS facilities could be contracted to the private sector, to provide investigations and appropriate diagnostic procedures.

Whilst it must also be recognised that 'freedom of choice' by both patients and professionals arise as an issue, this does not relate to equality of opportunity or a health care system based on need alone. To some extent, within a mixed system, health care policy will reflect the conflict between freedom of choice for the individual and that of equality of opportunity. Finally, because of the extensive cost of provision, the private sector will avoid dealing with chronic health care problems or crisis care, e.g. the long-term mentally ill, severely disabled and the chronically ill elderly person.

SUMMARY OF KEY POINTS

i)   Justice relates to equal distribution of and equal opportunity for health care and is one virtue amongst many

ii) The features of justice such as fairness (equity) and equality are not considered good in themselves but means of achieving ends

iii) It may be unjust when equal care and treatment is given if some people have greater needs

iv) Respect for persons is implicit in the two principles put forward by Rawls and his basic principle of justice is a notion of fairness (equity)

v)   The concepts of justice and fairness are not absolute virtues

vi) There should be distribution according to need not according to dessert

vii) The term equality is social, moral and prescriptive

viii) There is a requirement to respect persons equally when working for health care. This involves the requirement to respect autonomy in all people and comes from work establishing basic criteria for personhood

DISCUSSION QUESTIONS

1. How far is equality of health care concerned with justice and fairness?

2. If the concept of equality is used with regard to political aims, can health care provision ever be politically neutral?
3. How valuable is health care in relation to the pursuit of the good life?

4. How far can ethical issues be divorced from social issues when we claim that everyone has a right to health care? (The NHS exists through policy and legislation.)

5. Does everyone have a right to equal care and treatment?

6. What are the relevant inequalities that justify giving more to some and less to others?

7. Discuss the advantages and disadvantages of private health care.

Chapter 15
Preventive health care

Historically, within medicine itself there has been much more emphasis upon cure and treatment than on prevention and this relates to the allocation of resources.

While some health professionals, such as health visitors, have taken a central role in prevention and health promotion, some doctors have been resistant to such issues. However, many acknowledge that medical concern for potentially sick people may, in some situations, take priority over therapeutic medicine. (It is perhaps pertinent to mention that there are problems surrounding the history of the medical profession, its identity and education/training.)

Important factors for preventive health care include the resources available in the community and the differences between geographical areas. Issues concerning information given to the public and the way that information is related are involved. And prevention includes early diagnosis and screening.

The health of the community may conflict with the rights of an individual, e.g. in prevention of infectious diseases. Isolation of the person may be necessary to protect the rest of the community and this may impinge on the rights of the individual. It may also mean treatment when there is no sign of the disease. AIDS (Auto Immune Difficiency Syndrome) has raised even broader issues about the conflict between a person's health and prevention within the community. (There are problems for dentists and other health care workers.) The moral problems surround whether infective patients/clients/persons should be identified and whether those caring for them should be informed.

Major questions relating to implementation of rigorous preventive programmes surround: justifying infringing the liberty of the individual to improve the health of others; and the circumstances which should be taken into account when isolating, or placing restrictions on a person. (Remember that respect for persons is central to health ethics.)

Advertising and the transfer of information is important but how far should the doctor/health professional be involved in, say, stopping a person smoking without infringing individual freedom?

Prevention is the key to the control of many illnesses and several approaches can be used:

a) Alteration of life style: this involves attitudes, values and behaviour. There is a strong argument for doctors/health professionals to be educated in applied psychology and related ethical issues (AIDS, smoking, diet and exercise). There is some argument for attempting to change general public attitudes and values towards persons with infectious diseases

b) Identifying groups at high risk: this perhaps means following closely an individual's pattern of behaviour and trying to modify it in some way

c) Vaccination: this is widely used but there is always an element of risk, e.g. whooping cough vaccine

d) Screening: this makes sense and allows early diagnosis of a disease to be made, but problems may arise if false results are given

SUMMARY OF KEY POINTS

i) In medicine alone there has been much more emphasis upon cure than prevention

ii)   Important factors for preventive health include the resources that are available and the sort of information given to the public

iii)   Prevention includes early diagnosis and screening

iv)   Isolation of the person may be necessary to protect the rest of the community (by prevention)

v)   Prevention may involve justifying infringing the liberty of the individual

vi)   Different approaches can be used in preventive health care, e.g. changing life styles, identifying groups at high risk, vaccination and screening

DISCUSSION QUESTIONS

1. Why is the sort of information distributed to the public for preventive health important?

2. Preventive medicine relates to distribution of resources. What ethical issues arise when a judgement made is that prevention is better than cure?

3. What moral issues apply to decisions relating to screening procedures as a preventive method?

4. Do all members of the community have a right to preventive services?

5. Should the carers and the relatives of the person who carries an infectious disease be informed?

6. Should persons be informed if they are in high-risk categories and should they be allowed to refuse treatment?

5. Should the carers and the relatives of the person who carries an infectious disease be informed?

6. Should persons be informed if they are in high-risk categories and should they be allowed to refuse treatment?

Chapter 16
A study paper

A brief history of the conception of the nature of persons in relation to health care ethics

The authors make the assumption that understanding conceptions of persons is important in health care practice and subsequently respect for persons is central for applied ethics. A brief historical examination of selective views of the conception of the nature of persons will, therefore, encourage students to have a broader philosophical view. Understanding some of the ethical considerations and the philosophical contradictions that emerge is important, and in turn, this subsequently concerns views of whether the person should be analysed in terms of a single characteristic, a cluster of features or as a moral evaluative concept.

Concepts of the person, in philosophical terms that influence ethical issues, may roughly be divided between materialism and idealism (see Glossary of terms.) Further, what may be central for the nurse practitioner is whether persons are to be seen as active or passive. A commonsense view of the person also influences meaning within use, that is, how we use the term will influence the meaning we give to it (Henry, 1987). In other words, the concept of the person is as much a product of philosophical influence as individual and social consciousness.

HISTORICAL OVERVIEW

It seems sensible to proceed with a selective historical review of traditional philosophical ideas concerning the nature of persons in order to give some foundation on which to base the models presented in Chapter 5 and throughout the text. Traditionally, the mind has been seen as the central feature of the person and is one way of saying that persons are something quite different from other animals.

The person is perceived as more than a human being made of flesh and blood and this, indirectly, links with views about immortality of the spirit, mind and assertions about human dignity and free will. In turn, this links with views about personal autonomy and respect. The concept of a person is involved intimately with the notion of a being with a mind who can act freely, responsibly and morally. However, this is an ideal view (see Chapter 6, under Autonomy, p32).

Ancient Greek writers evolved influential theories incorporating psychophysical dualism (mind and body as separate entities). Both Socrates (469–399 BC) and Plato (428–348 BC) suggested a hierarchical structure of the person (Henry, 1986). The highest stratum of the mind was held to be reason; lower status was given to feelings and emotions and the lowest level in the hierarchical structure was designated for bodily features. According to Plato, a person's reason was the most important feature. Death was not an end in itself but an escape of the incorporate soul, emphasising the non-physical notion of soul or mind. For Plato, the real person was the soul or mind; this was the source of personal identity whereas the body was a shell and quite irrelevant.

Some modern theorists who take a more materialistic view have not inherited their views from Socrates or Plato but from Aristotle (384–322 BC), who presented a rather contrasting view and had a different approach to the nature of persons. Aristotle was a logician and biologist and opposed Plato's views. According to Aristotle, the person was a **composite** form made up of a psyche (translated as spirit) and matter.

Valentine (1982) suggests that Aristotle put forward a view of a **material** cause, a mechanistic explanation where reference is made to the physical embodiment of a system governing behaviour. The main feature of the person was reason (which governed action as well as intellect and knowledge gained) and was part of the **natural** world, not the **transcendental** world of Plato (part of the intellectual world of ideas not of the senses). Aristotle viewed persons as physical realities, which left little room for Platonic immorality, implying that the soul of a person was not separate from the body. Survival of persons after death rested upon an obscure capacity for abstract thought which did not involve any organ of the body. Further, this form did not show how individuality occurred without the body. Aristotle's doctrine recognised the importance of the external world and was the beginning of an interactionist account of the person that did not separate body and mind. According to Aristotle, what appeared to be essential was the identification of an individual body in the empirical reality of time and space.

Thomas Aquinas (1225 – 1274) not only developed Aristotlean concepts further but attempted to synthesise the two opposing metaphysical views put forward by Plato and Aristotle. Like Aristotle, Aquinas held that bodies individuated the differences between persons and they were seen to be different particles of matter. According to Aquinas, the intellect had the capacity to think, to form concepts and to possess beliefs, but the power to acquire ideas was achieved through sense experience, thereby emphasising the importance of interaction with the environment and the world. Other sentient beings such as other animals were seen to begin and end with birth and death respectively.

However, persons who had intellect and will (which belonged to the soul) remained after destruction of the body. In other words, a human person had a soul which, in life, was united with the body.

Much medieval philosophy centred on a dispute between Christian, Platonic and Aristotlean views. In very broad terms and with some qualifications it may be claimed that within more modern philosophical influences, this dispute has been replaced by rationalism and empiricism. Medieval philosophy shows how early influences still remain in the confusion that arises from separating the mind and body. The Platonic views emphasise the spiritual and rational considerations for caring for persons whilst Aristotle's and Aquinas' views emphasise the need to view the whole person in a more interactive way. Neither views give any answers but both lead to consideration of priorities in emphasis, particularly in health care, and recognise the person as active rather than passive. However, further philosophical influences highlight more contradictions between rationalism and empiricism. The rationalists views tend to highlight priorities of emphasis for personal autonomy and responsibility, whereas empiricism, if taken too literally, could link indirectly, not only to a medical model, but to viewing the person as mechanistic and perhaps passive. However, caution is needed in making any broad generalisations. What is essential is to broaden the nurse practitioner's philosophical understanding of the problems and subsequently, provide more reflective ways of understanding practical ethical issues about caring for persons.

The intellectual nature of the person inherited dualistic notions and was given force by Plato, moderated by Aristotle, entangled with Aquinas and developed into a rational position of **classical dualism** by René Descartes (1596–1650).

Descartes separated mind and body and the idea of the subjective self emerged by having a non-physical mind. Descartes belonged to the Platonic tradition in that he considered the soul or mind, by its very nature, to be totally independent of the body. Bodies of persons could be seen as machines governed entirely by the laws of physics. Descartes drew a sharp distinction between persons and animals because the former had minds. According to Descartes it was inconceivable that any material mechanism could think (Flew, 1964). The problem is that persons are also physical beings in a physical universe. However, the tendency to separate mind and body remains with us and is evident in the confusions that arise in conceptualising what we mean by being a person and subsequently, respect for persons in health care.

Mind has the distinguishing features of thoughts and feelings whereas the body can have form, motion and causal interactions described by physical laws (as described in applied biology, physiology and so on).

Persons do have special access to their own individual mental states without gathering data by observation or from the physical state of the body. This view of subjective self-knowledge not only encompasses the Cartesian psychological view about the self but also relates to the view of higher-order attributes assigned to a concept of a rational mind which is a central feature of the person. Do we conceive of the person as having one major characteristic, i.e. that of a rational mind and is that what distinguishes persons from non-persons?

The doctrine of Immanuel Kant (1724–1804) is complex and deserves more than the cursory overview given here. However, it is essential to encapsulate at least some of his central ideas of persons that are generally supportive of a moral and evaluative use of the term person. His doctrine also arose out of the **rationalism** of Descartes and the **empiricism** of Locke, Berkeley and Hume. Kant opposed Locke's view of the mind being a *tabula rasa* (a smooth tablet upon which impressions of the external events imprint themselves) in claiming that the mind was not passive but active. He believed the person had control over his or her thoughts and actions. However, according to Kant, we cannot see the external world independently of our human way of knowing (being human implies that we are in a physical/sensory universe). Kant saw the human mind as active, ordering the raw material of sense experience into a world of conceptualised phenomena. The connectedness of our perceptions is viewed as produced by the activity of mind (Strawson, 1959).

According to Henry (1986), Kant reflects a **phenomeno- logical** approach and Valentine (1982) suggests that this approach avoids dualism between subjective and objective, and the reduction of one to another which, in turn, avoids extreme rationalism and the over-emphasis of the rational mind as the necessary central feature of a person. Further, it avoids over-emphasis of empiricism and in turn can be expressed as emphasising the agent/person's perspective and the meaning of a situation for the person.

Kant claims cause and effect to work within a physical world; hence, persons or more specifically physical bodies are subject to causal relations. Nevertheless, cause and effect cannot affect human reason and persons are rational in that they can exercise free thought and action. According to Kant, free will is a self regulator and, in turn, the person can impose laws upon itself. Rational beings should act so that his/her actions conform to universal laws (see Chapter 8, Two major perspectives of morality). A law yields what Kant termed a **categorical imperative**. A law which operates and applies to one's self should operate and apply to all rational beings. It is here that moral laws derive from rationality (see Chapter 8, under Kantian ethics).

In summary, Kant defines the person as a rational being with an active mind and capable of imposing laws upon him/herself; worthy of respect. From the Kantian perspective, that which gives a person absolute worth is his or her possession of a rational will. These notions of the ability to choose for oneself, to be self-determined, having practical ability, moral responsibility and free will are essential attributes of persons. Kant, and later Strawson (1959), have convincingly argued that we can only identify mental states of spatially located persons.

It is perhaps essential to discuss briefly selective alternatives which reflect more monist and materialistic views. Puzzlement about the nature of mental states encourages alternative explanations that have been influential for our conception of persons.

So far, the traditional philosophers have either referred to recognising one major characteristic of persons, that is the mind, or alternatively, a cluster of features of the person. Gilbert Ryle (1900–1976) criticised Cartesian dualism and referred to the mind, i.e. the invisible entity inhabiting the body, as the 'ghost in the machine'. Ryle believed that the mind did not lie behind but within behaviour. He reduced the self to a bundle of dispositions and behaviour. Mind and matter were not different substances; only mental and physical concepts (or ideas) were different (**conceptual dualism**).

Behaviour and performance were important criteria for recognising persons. The person was viewed as a higher form of mammal. According to Ryle the term person could well be viewed as a social notion in that persons display behaviour and only have being within the social context. Infants and idiots did not have minds because they did not have complicated dispositions so were not viewed as full persons. The question arises: can we unhook dispositions from inner features and intentions of the agent? Behaviourism does not allow us to recognise such inner lives.

J.C.C. Smart's theory (1959) of central state materialism maintains that the human being is a vast arrangement of physical particles, and that states of consciousness are only behavioural facts about the mechanism and sensations of the brain. The person is distinguishable from a non-human animal by differences in brain size and complexity of brain processes. Nevertheless, since it is possible that a non-human person could exist in the universe who did not have a physiological make-up similar to ourselves, with no organ that could be clearly identified as a brain, then it would be wrong to claim that personal identity counts as brain identity.

Strawson (1959) claims that the concept of the person is primitive and unanalysable, and that what he calls personal predicates, i.e. both states of consciousness and corporeal characteristics, can be ascribed to persons. However, we already assume from this perspective what a person is. None of the philosophical views so far can give any satisfactory answer and they must be viewed only as different conceptual schemes that may or may not widen our understanding as practitioners of care. The next three modern philosophical views may help to broaden our understanding further, particularly within the health care domain.

THREE MODERN VIEWS

Abelson maintained in 1977 that person status cannot be proved at all because we do not have established criteria for applying person status to other animals or machines. Nevertheless, we might apply the status of person to non-humans, particularly if they are strikingly like us in appearance. (Some animals such as the chimpanzee show a strong resemblance.)

It is really open to us whether we ascribe person status to them or not and neither logic nor language can tell us which animals should and which should not be given the title person. Abelson also claims that even if we find grounds in the behaviour of others for calling them persons, behaviour alone does not entail granting such status. Abelson claims that the giving of person status does not rest entirely on respect for human beings since the mental defective or the very small infant are human beings but are often given semi-person status. Similarly, in recent social history a whole race of human beings were deprived of full person status (the Jews in Nazi Germany).

Abelson refers to the term person as an evaluative term, resembling the moral term good. It is open-ended and cannot be analysed empirically. According to Abelson the person is a subject of both psychological and moral predicates and is independent of biological classification; therefore it is possible to ascribe person status to non-humans. The term person is viewed as normative and evaluative rather than descriptive (see Chapter 1, Introduction and Chapter 5, Persons). It is not a necessary truth that all person are human beings.

Locke (1632–1704) distinguishes between the identity of a person and that of a man, holding that the latter does, while the former does not, involve the identity of an animal (Swinborne, 1984). Swinborne remarks that the animal is that in which the person is physically realised at a given time. However, Abelson, like Kant and Strawson, concludes that the body is essential for identification of persons in a physical universe.

Daniel Dennett, in 1979, developed further the features and content of persons, and outlined some possible themes that have been identified as necessary, but on their own not sufficient, conditions for being a person. He claims that the idea of an intelligent conscious feeling agent coincides with the moral notion of the person who is accountable, having rights and responsibilities. It is, therefore, necessary to have an intelligent conscious and feeling agent in order to have a moral notion of a person. This assumption supports and underpins a Kantian view of morality deriving from rationality (see Chapter 8, Two major perspectives of morality).

Dennett suggests that the most obvious condition is that persons are viewed as rational and this links closely to some of the traditional views of persons put forward by Plato, Aristotle, Kant and others. Reason also involves higher-order notions of knowledge, language and intelligence. Secondly, states of consciousness are attributed to persons and we give intentions to them. Thirdly, something counting as a person rests upon a particular attitude or stance being adopted. In other words, individuals are treated in a certain way and this, to some extent, is constitutive of being a person. The fourth point is reciprocity, by which we mean that a being who has a particular stance taken towards it must reciprocate in some way. The fifth point involves communication and the sixth indicates that a special kind of consciousness emerges, i.e. self-consciousness which, in turn, is a condition for persons being moral agents.

Dennett's themes identify a common cluster of features but he points out that his view is an ideal notion of the nature of persons which would be difficult, if not impossible, to apply in certain cases (e.g. six-month-old foetus, mentally handicapped person, demented elderly person).

Finally, Jenny Teichman in 1972, adopted a Wittgenstein approach and this can be developed into what we could call a commonsense view of the person (see Henry, 1986). According to Teichman in commonsense terms we treat humanity as the deciding factor when ascribing personhood. It may be assumed that in commonsense terms the use of the term human means two things: being a member of a species and being a person (see Chapter 5, Persons). Teichman suggests that the extension of the term human being gives the impression that these two things are identical. She also claims that both in law and in theology use of the term human being is a starting point for the term person. The only actual persons we meet in real life are human beings although it is logically possible for the existence of other varieties of natural persons on other planets (non-human persons).

Teichman's view relates to Wittgenstein's approach in that language is seen as essentially social. The meaning of a word is not to be found by logical analysis but in its use within the particular language game to which it belongs. These language games are not just a matter of words and use but also include feelings, gestures, attitudes and skills. Wittgenstein claimed that these complex related elements compose a particular form of life and language used in each game overlaps, sharing the same words but having different meanings. Crudely, it can be illustrated in the use of the word human. In one particular language game, in a dialogue between biologists,human may be used to mean biological membership of a species whereas in another language game between nurses it can be used in the same way as the word person.

The central point is our conceptions of persons will be influenced to some extent by the commonsense meaning and general use of the word. Language functions in both social and professional contexts.

Footnote

Hopefully this study paper will provoke thought in relation to the conceptions of persons and subsequently respect for persons held to be central to health care and underpinning ethical concerns for actions and decisions made within the health care and nursing domains.

Chapter 17
Glossary of terms

Absolutism: The view that moral standards are valid universally and that their content and authority does not vary according to the circumstances (cf. relativism)

Altruism (ethical): The view that morality requires greater weight being given to other people's welfare than to one's own, (cf. egoism)

Analytic: Statements are necessary (necessarily true) e.g. triangles have three sides. True on logical as opposed to factual or empirical grounds. Truly a apriori. (Statements which are not analytic are known as synthetic)

A *posteriori* statement: A statement of which the truth or falsity can only be ascertained empirically (by observation or experiment). These sorts of statements are consequently synthetic and contingent

Autonomy of ethics: That moral terms, such as good, right and ought, cannot be defined purely descriptively or factually and moral judgements cannot be deduced from premises which do not include moral judgements. Generally, most upholders of autonomy of ethics maintain that morality is a subject in its own right and cannot be reduced to science, religion or custom

Categorical imperative: The Kantian principle that one ought never to act except on a maxim that can be willed as a universal law, e.g. promises ought to be kept. Categorical imperatives are not conditional.

Glossary of terms

Concept: A person who understands the terms 'good', 'free', 'person', 'triangle' or 'red' may be said to have the concepts of good, free, person, triangle or red. Philosophy, which is greatly concerned with the meaning of terms and the logical relationships between the statements, is said to be a **conceptual** enquiry as opposed to a factual enquiry

Contingent: Not necessary (empirical statements are contingent)

Deontological theory An enquiry into the nature of moral duty and rightness of actions

Determinism: Any view according to which all actions are caused, predictable in principle and explicable according to scientific laws. Free-will problems involve whether or not actions which are in some way determined can also be free. (This is relevant for moral responsibility.)

Dualism: A theory concerned with individuals being divided into two substances, either material or mental, both of which cannot be regarded as part of the other

Duty (moral): An act held to be morally obligatory (see Chapter 8, under Kantian ethics, p48)

Egoism (ethical): The view that morality requires or permits one to set more importance by one's own welfare than that of other people. Ethical egoism is to be distinguished from psychological egoism, which maintains not that people should or may, but that they do prefer their own welfare to that of any others (cf. altruism)

Emotive meaning: Aspects of the meaning of a word expressing emotion or attitude rather than communicating factual information

Emotivism: The view that moral judgements are exclusively for expression of emotions or attitudes

Empiricism: The thesis that all knowledge of matters of fact is based upon experience. It rejects Platonism and idealism.

Ethics: Sometimes this can mean the same as moral philosophy; at other times it refers to parts of the subject matter of moral philosophy

Evaluative: This is to be distinguished from descriptive or factual meaning. Prescriptivism and emotivism are different accounts of evaluative meaning

Exculpation, excuse: A person will not be held culpable for doing something. (Exculpate – remove guilt altogether). Health worries might be held to excuse a person for neglect of responsibilities

Hypothetical imperative: The opposite to the categorical imperative, e.g. If you want X do Y, Y being the means to achieving X

Idealism: A name given to a group of philosophical theories having a common view that the external world is created by the mind

Locution: Used in text as a general word for referring to both factual statements and moral judgements. Cannot be used in ordinary language because some philosophers do not believe that moral judgements are statements

Logic: The systematic study of the rules of valid arguments and all related matters. Logical viewpoints contrast with moral and factual statements, e.g. a triangle has three sides – logic; in Australia some swans are black – factual; racial discrimination is morally bad – moral

Materialism: The belief that whatever exists is either matter or entirely dependent upon matter for existence

Naturalism (ethical): Any view according to which moral judgements can be seen as factual or empirical

Naturalistic fallacy: This occurs when moral words like 'good', 'right' or 'ought' are defined purely factually or descriptively, or when they are deducible from factual statements. (See G. Moore and Utilitarianism when 'good' equals 'happiness'.)

Glossary of terms

Necessary condition: This is a premise which must be true in order to reach a certain conclusion (cf sufficient condition), for example having four sides is a necessary condition for being square (but a figure with four sides need not necessarily be square). See Dennett's necessary but not sufficient conditions for personhood, (Henry, 1986)

Normative: This is generally concerned with rules and recommendations as contrasted to description. It implies a norm of standard and value.

Objectivism: Any view to which moral judgements are statements about something other than the agent's state of mind (cf. subjectivism and objectivism).

Other regarding: Caring for others besides oneself and, therefore, valuing others and ensuring they have rights and respect accorded to them as persons

Positivism (moral): Any view which identifies morality with a current social code, e.g. simple rules or codes of conduct

Predicate: This belongs to Aristotlean logic. It is that which is affirmed or denied of the subject, for example the rational mind is predicated to the person

Prescriptivism: A view where moral judgements have some important affinities with imperatives or commands (see Kant)

Rationalism: A doctrine of a group of 17th and 18th century philosophers who believed that it was possible to obtain knowledge of what exists by reason. For example, Descartes: *Cogito ergo sum* – I think therefore I am

Rawls' hypothetical situation: Rawls based his two principles upon a hypothetical situation. We should imagine a group of people coming together who were separated from their own personalities and situations by a veil of ignorance. They would not know, therefore, if they were young, old, black, white, male, female, talented or stupid. (We have no experience of this so it remains hypothetical)

Relativism The view that knowledge is of our own relations with the outside world only. (Opposite to absolutism)

Sufficient condition: A premise which, if true, means that the conclusion must also be true. For example, if a shape is a square, it must have four sides

Transcendental: Any theory that asserts that the world is based upon the mind and is activities of reason

Universalisability: A feature of moral judgements by virtue of which anyone who holds that someone ought to do a certain thing is committed to holding that everyone in similar circumstances ought to act in a similar way

Utilitarianism: The view that morality is or should be based upon the principle of utility – the greatest happiness of the greatest number. (See Chapter 8, under Utilitarianism,p42–44)

Chapter 18
Bibliography and recommended reading

Abelson, R. (1977). *Persons: A study in Philosophical Psychology*, Macmillan, London

Benjamin, M. and Curtis, J. (1981). *Ethics in Nursing*, Oxford University Press

Benn, S.I. and Peters, R.S. (1975). *Social Principles and the Democratic State*, George Allen & Unwin

Dennett, D. (1979). *Brainstorms*, Harvester Press, Sussex

Downie, R.S. and Calman, K.C. (1987). *Health Respect: Ethics in Health Care*, Faber & Faber, London

Fitzpatrick, F.J. (1988). *Ethics in Nursing Practice*, The Linacre Centre, London

Flew, A. (1964). *Body, Mind and Death*, Macmillan

Flew, A. (1979). *A Dictionary of Philosophy*, Pan Books, London

Fried, C. (1970). *An Anatomy of Values*, Harvard University Press

Geach, P.T. (1976). *Reason and Arguments*, Blackwell, London

Gillon, R. (1985). *Philosophical Medical Ethics*, John Wiley & Sons

Glover, J. (1972). *Responsibility*, Routledge and Kegan Paul

Hanfling, O. (1978). *Fundamental Problems of Philosophy*, Oxford University Press

Hare, R.M. (1987). *Invitro Fertilisation, Ethics and Reproduction and Genetic Control*, ed. R. Chadwick, p.71-89, Routledge

Harris, J. (1985). *The Value of Life*, Routledge & Kegan Paul, London

Hampshire, S. (1959). *Thoughts and Action*, Chatto Windus, London

Henry, I.C. (1986). *The Concept of the Person*, Unpublished PhD thesis, Leeds University

Henry, I.C. and Tuxill, A.C. (1987). Conceptions of persons: An introduction to health care professionals' curriculum. *J. Adv. Nursing*, **12**, 245–249

Henry, I.C. and Tuxill, A.C. (1987). Persons and humans, *J. Adv. Nursing*, **12**, 383–388

Hospers, J. (1973). *An Introduction to Philosophical Analysis*, Routledge & Kegan Paul, London

Joad, C.E.M. (1977). *Philosophy (19th edn.)*, Hodder & Stoughton

Magee, B.(ed.) (1978). *Men of Ideas*, British Broadcasting Corporation

Midgley, M. (1983). *Animals and Why They Matter*, Penguin Books, Harmondsworth

Mill, J.S. (1977), *Utilitarianism*, Penguin

Popper, K.P. (1966). *The Open Society and its Enemies, 5th edn.*, Routledge and Kegan Paul

Rand, A. (1964). *The Virtue of Selfishness*, American Library, New York

Russell, B. (1974). *History of Western Philosophy*, George Allen & Unwin, London

Singer, P. (1986). *Applied Ethics*, Oxford University Press

Strawson, P.F. (1959). *Individuals*, Methuen

Swinborne, S. and Shoemaker, R. (1984). *Personal Identity*, Basil Blackwell

Teichman, J. (1985). The definition of person, *J. R. Inst. Phil.*, **60**, 175–185

Telfer, A. (1980). *Caring and Caring*, Methuen

Thiroux, J. (1977). *Ethics*, Glenco Publishers, London

Valentine, E. (1982). *Conceptual Issues in Psychology*, George Allen & Unwin.

Warnock, M. (1977). *Schools of Thought*, Faber & Faber, London

Wilson, B.R. (ed.) (1975). *Education, Equality and Society*, George Allen & Unwin

Index